Down Syndrome and Other Chromosome Abnormalities

Edited by Subrata Kumar Dey

Published in London, United Kingdom

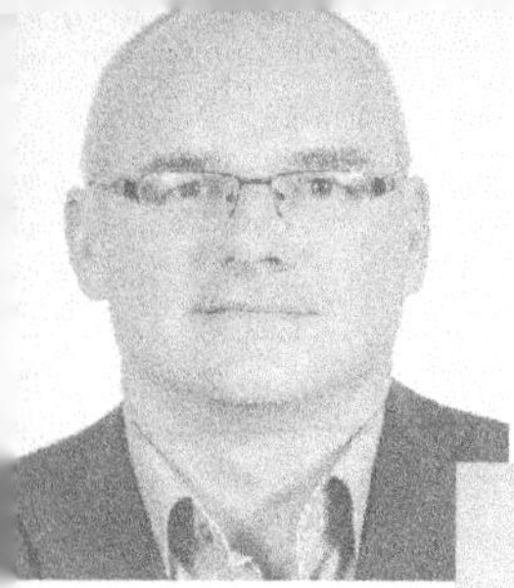
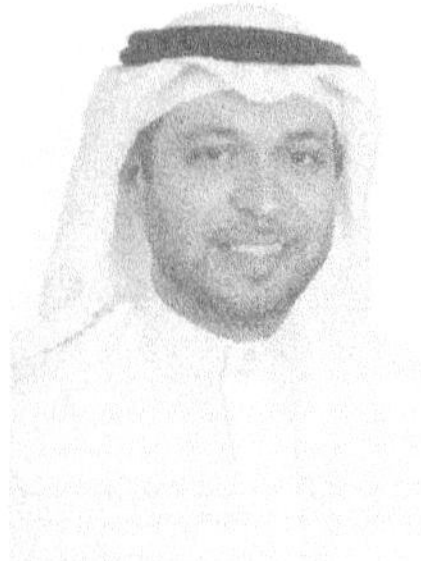
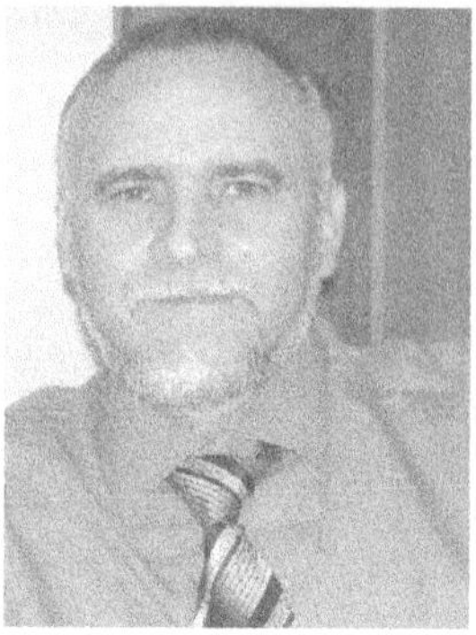
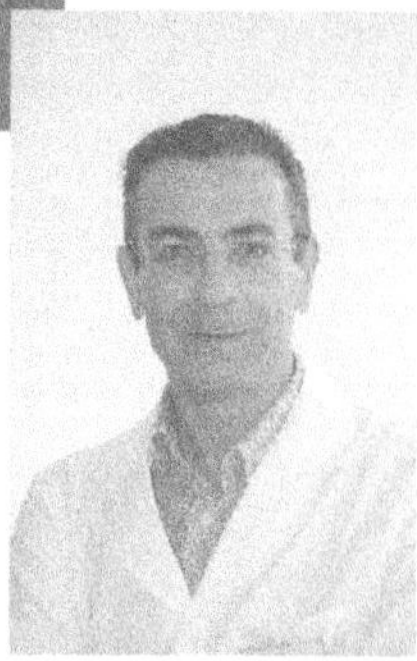
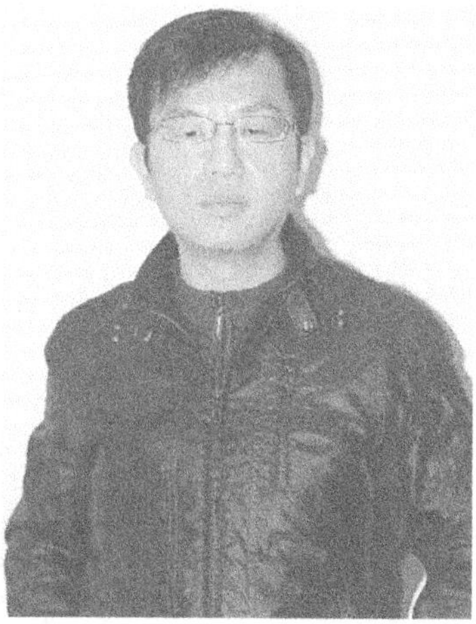
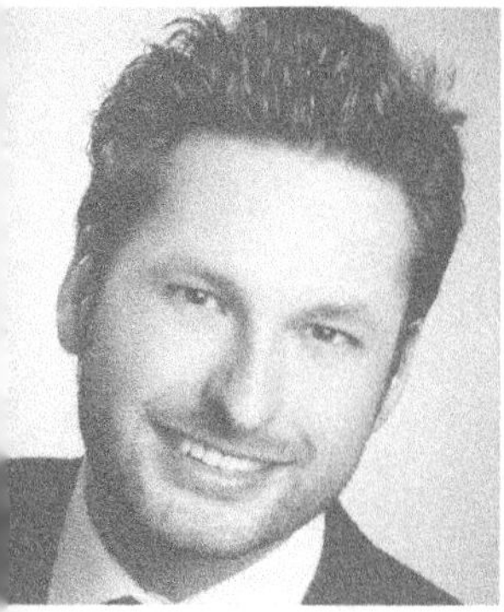
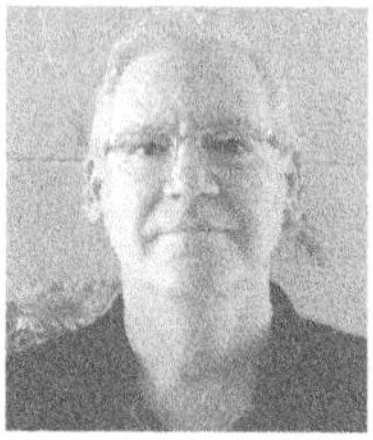

IntechOpen

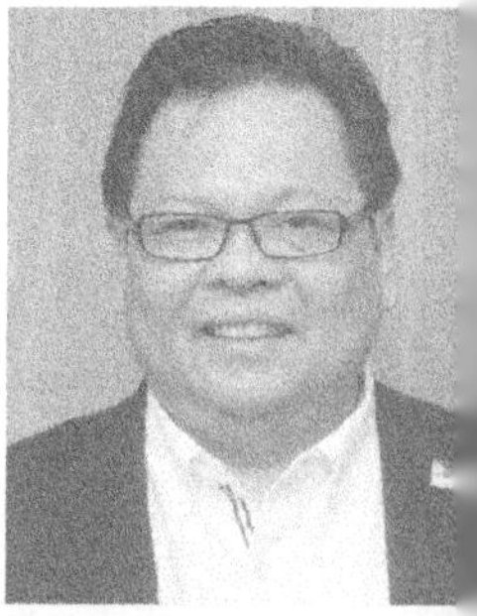
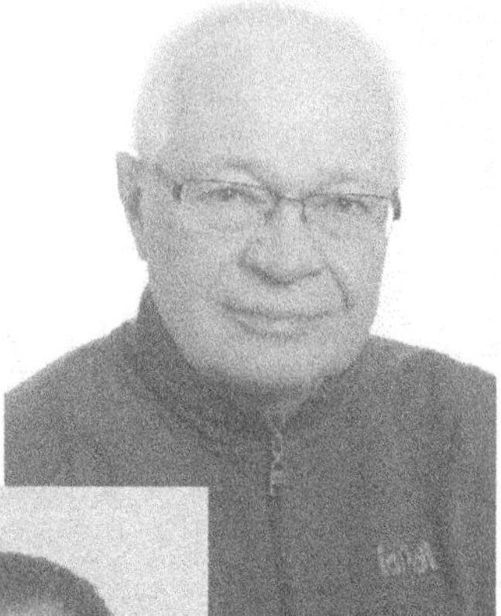
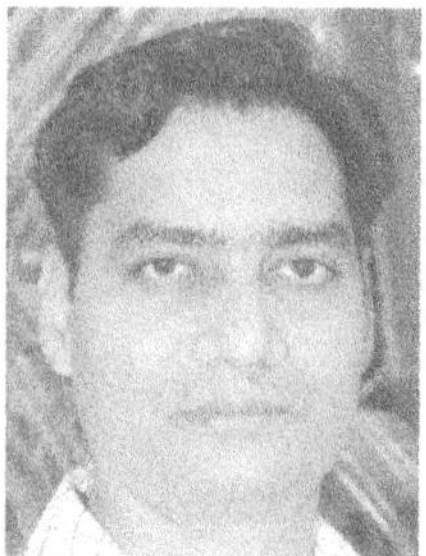
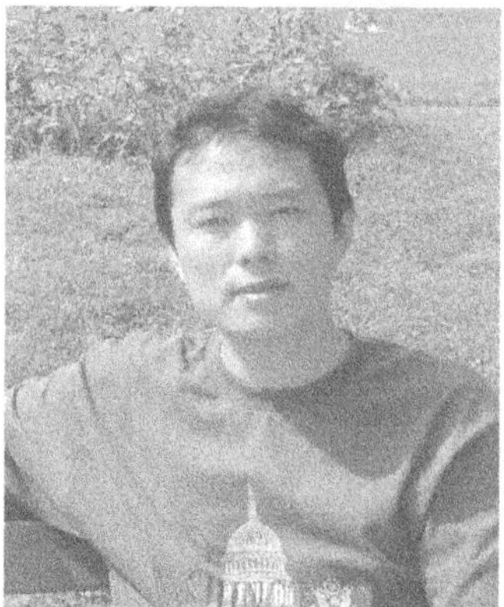
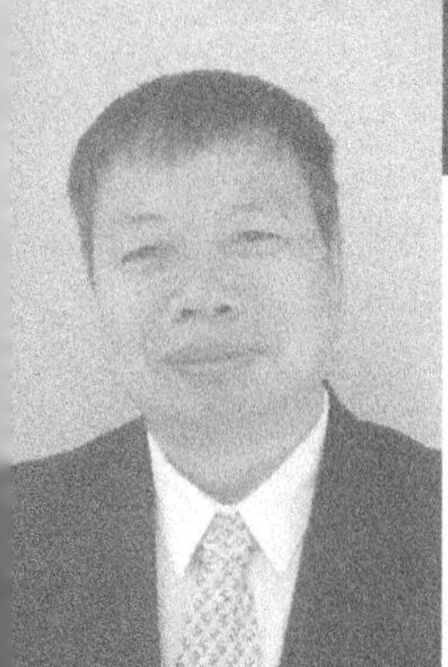
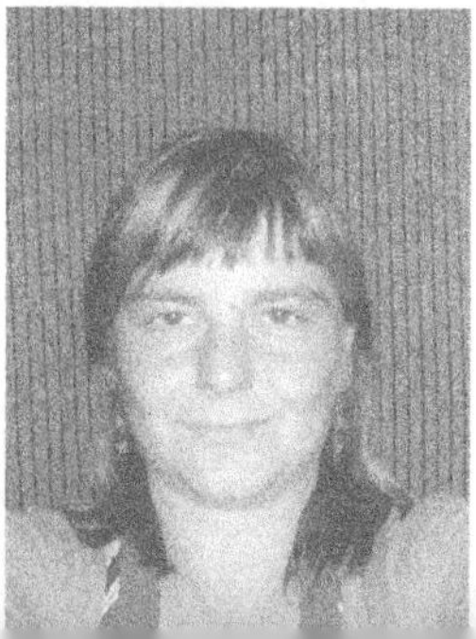

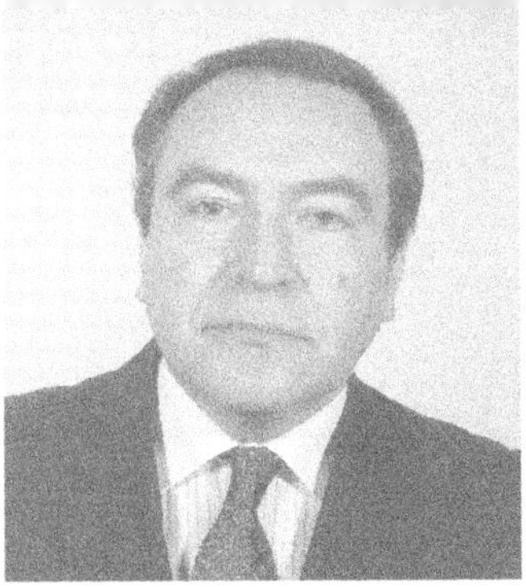

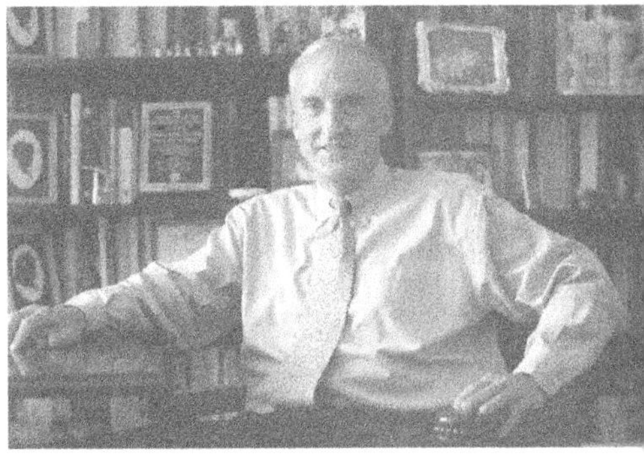

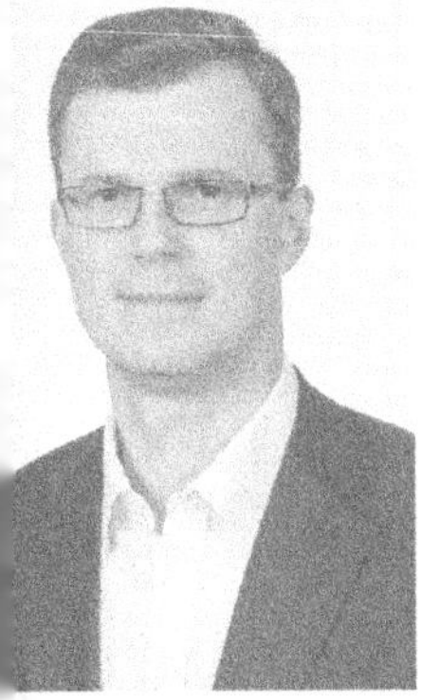

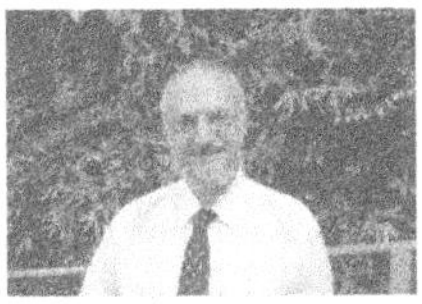

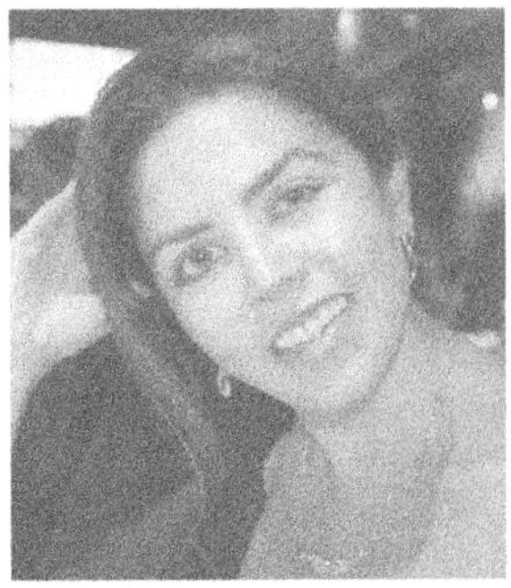

Supporting open minds since 2005

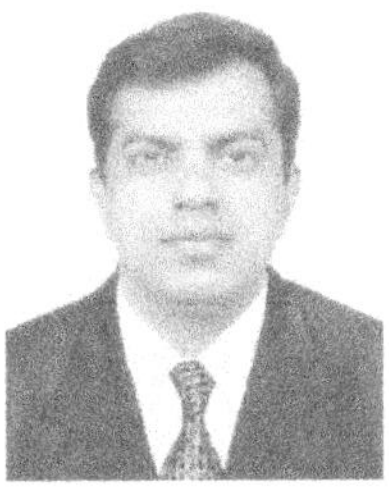

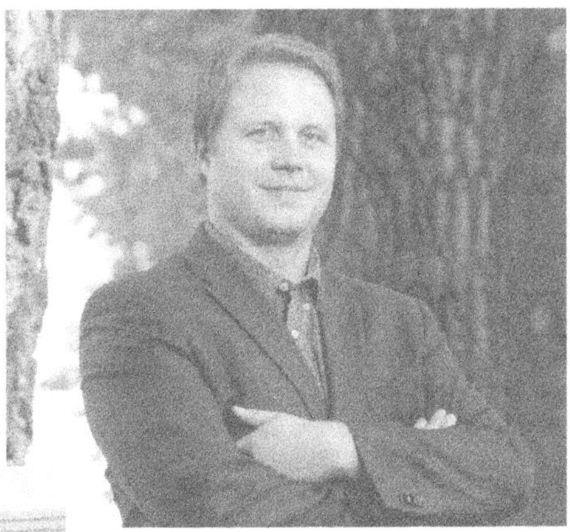

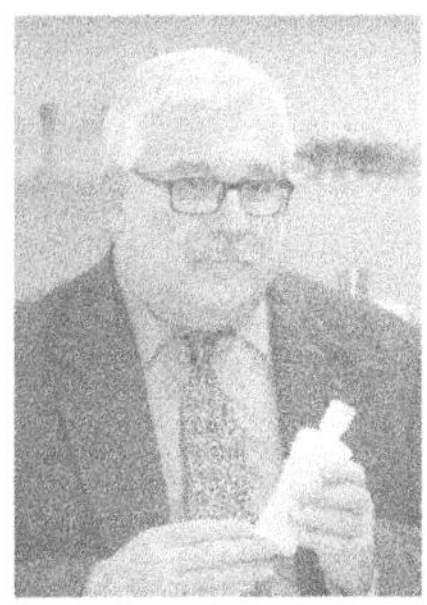

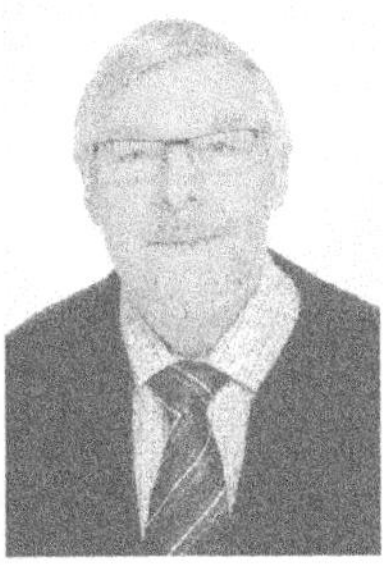

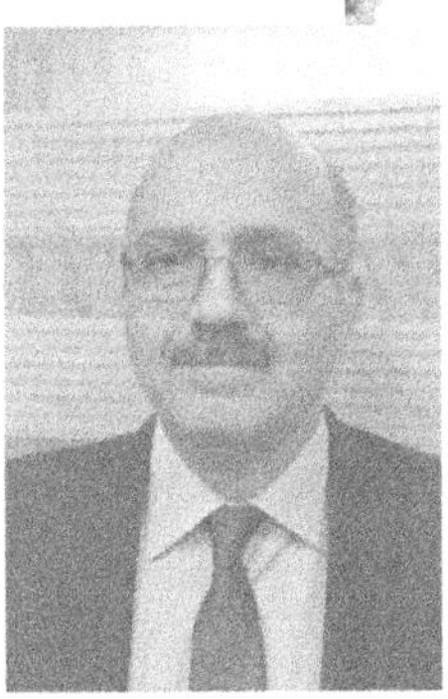

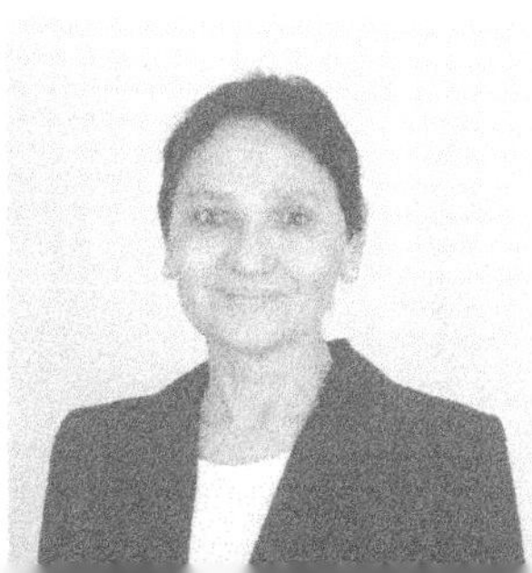

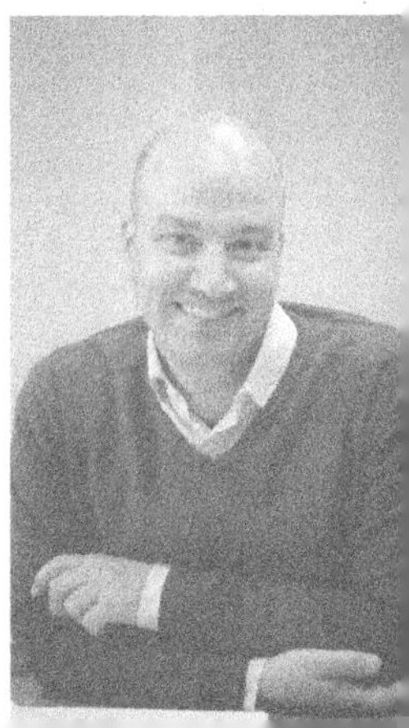

Down Syndrome and Other Chromosome Abnormalities
http://dx.doi.org/10.5772/intechopen.91519
Edited by Subrata Kumar Dey

Contributors
Emine Ikbal Atli, Zainab Al-Suhaymi, Fatma Söylemez, Madhavilatha Routhu, Shiva Surya Varalakshmi Koneru, Subhadra Poornima, Saranya Vadrevu, Imran Ali Khan, Hariharan Sreedharan, Van Hieu Van Pham, Subrata Kumar Dey, Poulami Majumder

First published in London, United Kingdom, 2022 by IntechOpen
IntechOpen is the global imprint of INTECHOPEN LIMITED, registered in England and Wales, registration number: 11086078, 5 Princes Gate Court, London, SW7 2QJ, United Kingdom
Printed in Croatia

British Library Cataloguing-in-Publication Data
A catalogue record for this book is available from the British Library

Additional hard and PDF copies can be obtained from orders@intechopen.com

Down Syndrome and Other Chromosome Abnormalities
Edited by Subrata Kumar Dey
p. cm.
Print ISBN 978-1-83969-364-9
Online ISBN 978-1-83969-365-6
eBook (PDF) ISBN 978-1-83969-366-3

Meet the editor

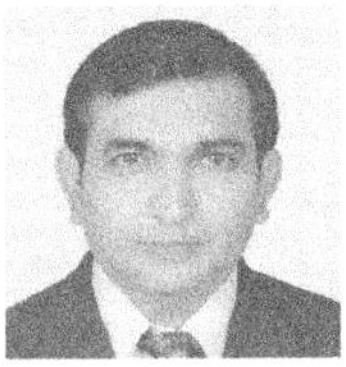

Professor Subrata Kumar Dey, Ph.D., vice-chancellor, Swami Vivekananda University, West Bengal, India, has been associated with teaching and research for more than four decades and had visited different countries as an invited speaker to deliver lectures. He was a professor of biotechnology at the Maulana Abul Kalam Azad University of Technology, West Bengal, India, and was director of the School of Biotechnology and Biological Sciences, West Bengal, India. His laboratory had long been involved in research on the molecular genetics of Down syndrome, congenital heart disease and Alzheimer disease. He published more than a hundred research papers, edited several books on Down syndrome and had completed eleven research projects. Several students obtained Ph.D. under his supervision. Along with teaching and research, Professor Dey handled a number of administrative assignments successfully and had made dedicated and innovative approaches with great integrity. His major administrative roles were director of Centre for Genetic Studies and pro-vice-chancellor and vice-chancellor, Maulana Abul Kalam Azad University of Technology, India.

Contents

Preface

Accurate diagnosis of a specific congenital disorder is a necessary prerequisite in providing a prognosis and plan of management for the affected infant. The development of a reliable technique for chromosome analysis led to the discovery of several chromosomal syndromes. Karyotype provides a complete genomic profile of individual diploid chromosomal characteristics. It reveals changes in chromosome numbers and structures. The numerical change in the autosome is the cause of Down syndrome or trisomy 21. This is the most common genetic cause of mental retardation and the most frequent autosomal trisomies among liveborns. In approximately 95% of cases, the extra chromosome 21 occurs as a result of meiotic nondisjunction or abnormal segregation of chromosomes. The risk factors associated with the development of Down syndrome are enigmatic. The overall maternal risk factors that cause Down syndrome are multifactorial and include both genetic and environmental factors. The changes in the number of sex chromosomes result in Turner, Klinefelter and other sex chromosomal abnormality syndromes, while structural changes in the chromosome, such as deletion, duplication and translocation, are also responsible for different types of chromosomal disorders. These abnormalities account for a large proportion of spontaneous pregnancy loss and childhood disability. It also contributes to the genesis of a significant proportion of malignancy in both childhood and adult life.

This book is organized into five sections and all sections include chapters that focused on recent scientific advancements in research on Down syndrome and other chromosomal abnormality syndromes and diseases associated with these disorders. The editor endeavoured to consistently use scientific terminology in review articles to keep the original text intact.

The first section includes the introductory chapter where the author has highlighted recent advancements in research on Down syndrome, different types of syndromes due to numerical and structural alterations of chromosomes and the role of prenatal diagnosis in the management of these congenital disorders.

The second section deals with the origin and mechanisms of aneuploidy, the role of polyploidy in evolution and the impact of climate change on genetic alteration.

The third section focuses on the effect of sociodemographic factors on different congenital disorders, causes of Down syndrome and phenotype associated with Down syndrome.

The fourth section covers haematological malignancies, congenital heart disease and surgical intervention in Down syndrome.

The concluding section discusses prenatal screening and management and genetic counselling to detect Down syndrome and other chromosomal abnormalities.

The editor wants to acknowledge the superb assistance of the staff members and management of IntechOpen in particular Mrs. Dolores Kuzelj for the coordination and editorial assistance. I am grateful to all the contributing authors and scientists who made this book possible by providing valuable research and review articles.
Finally, I would like to dedicate this book to the children with Down syndrome and other congenital disorders who need our love and care to lead a healthy life.

Subrata Kumar Dey
Swami Vivekananda University,
West Bengal, India

Section 1

Introduction

Chapter 1

Introductory Chapter: Down Syndrome and Other Chromosome Abnormalities

Subrata Kumar Dey

1. Introduction

Down syndrome (DS) is one of the most frequent autosomal disorders in humans and is also known as trisomy 21. Its incidence at birth is approximately 1 in 700 [1–3]. Down syndrome is associated with mental retardation, typical facial appearance, congenital heart disease, leukemia, gastrointestinal malformation, Alzheimer's disease, and several other congenital abnormalities with varying degree of severity [4]. Investigation on DS karyotype revealed a diploid chromosome number of 2n = 47, XX/XY, +21 in 95% cases, while mosaicism was found in approximately 2% of cases. On the other hand, Robertsonian translocations involving 13q21q or 14q21q or 21q21q account for approximately 3% of all DS cases [5].

Mental retardation is one of the most important clinical features of Down syndrome. Interests were generated to understand the cause of mental retardation among DS live births and to explore the etiology of Down syndrome. Genotyping using polymorphic microsatellite markers had enabled the investigators [6, 7] to study the maternal meiotic errors and also to look into the candidate genes responsible for DS pathophysiology. Two established risk factors for the birth of DS babies are advanced maternal age [8] and altered recombination [9]. Study of parental origin of extra chromosome 21, stage of meiotic nondisjunction, and recombination pattern revealed the overall reduction in meiotic recombination irrespective of maternal age [3, 10].

Human chromosome 21 (HC21) is one of the smallest acrocentric chromosomes. Investigation revealed that 21q22 contains genes in triplicated condition, which are responsible for DS phenotype. This segment was regarded as Down Syndrome Critical Region (DSCR) [4, 11]. After the completion of sequencing of HC21, several genes and their prospective functions had been identified. Triplication and overexpression of which significantly contributed toward the development of DS phenotype [12, 13].

Besides advanced maternal age, environmental risk factors for the birth of DS babies have also been identified, which include smokeless chewing tobacco, oral contraceptives [14], and cigarette smoking [15]. However, there was lack of convincing evidence regarding risk of maternal drinking during gestational period for DS births [16].

Though advanced maternal age is one of the most important risk factors for the meiotic nondisjunction of chromosome 21 in DS individuals, investigation of this association at the genetic level, involving telomere length measurement, is still limited [17]. Measurement of telomere length in older mothers with DS babies revealed shorter telomere than age-matched control mothers without DS babies. It has been suggested that older mothers with DS babies are genetically older than control euploid

IntechOpen

mother, and telomere length attrition or genetic aging may be associated with nondisjunction of chromosome 21 during first and second meiotic divisions [10].

Mouse has been used extensively for genetic experiment and also to study any human chromosomal alterations. The rapid development of genetic engineering provided the impetus for the generation of multiple Down syndrome mouse models in order to better understand the pathophysiology and also to correlate genotype with the phenotype in DS. Two segmental mouse models in widely use are Ts65Dn [18] and Ts1Cje [19, 20]. Moreover, the discovery of new editing technology CRISPR/Cas9 DNA repairing processes has facilitated the development of new therapeutic strategies to cure human genetic diseases and associated chromosomal abnormalities [21].

Besides mental retardation, DS individuals are also affected by multiple diseases. Congenital heart defect such as atrioventricular septal defect (AVSD) is prevalent among 40–60% of DS individuals [22]. Further investigation on AVSD revealed that there is an association between CRELD1 gene and AVSD in DS and euploid individuals [23]. A growing body of evidence shows that a major portion of DS population acquires Alzheimer's Disease, such as neuropathological changes by the age of 55–60 years, and develops dementia [24]. Recent studies [25] revealed that there is a close association between Alzheimer's disease and Down syndrome, and this may be due to the fact that they also share common genetic risk factors. Two genes, Presenilin-1 (PSEN-1) and Apolipoprotein E (APOE), are found to be associated with early- and late- onset Alzheimer's disease in Down syndrome. On the other hand, the incidence of acute leukemia (AL) is very high in children with Down syndrome (70–100%) compared with children without this syndrome. Among the children with DS who develop leukemia, 60% is classified as having acute lymphoblastic leukemia (ALL) and 40% with acute myeloblastic leukemia (AML) [26].

Recent studies on the infection with COVID-19 virus show that DS patients are at increased risk for death from infection with the virus since the DS patients are associated with dysfunction of immune system, congenital heart disease, and pulmonary pathology [27].

2. Other chromosome syndromes

Down syndrome is the most frequent autosomal abnormality and shows a strong association with advanced maternal age and reduced recombination. With advancement of our knowledge on diagnostic procedures such as karyotyping, fluorescence *in situ* hybridization (FISH) and molecular diagnosis involving microsatellite markers result in the recognition of an increasing number of new chromosome abnormalities, which include both numerical and structural chromosomal aberrations. Though on an individual basis these disorders are rare in occurrence, together they account for a loss of very high proportion of human conceptions. To date, well over 100 chromosome syndromes have been reported [5]. Most of these disorders are either autosomal or sex chromosomal in origin, while a small percentage of such patients have a structural chromosome abnormalities such as deletion, duplication, or translocation. Here, we have discussed some common chromosomal syndromes.

Edward's syndrome or trisomy 18 where there is a nondisjunction of chromosome no. 18. Most trisomic 18 individuals die in embryonic or fetal stage [28], while nondisjunction of chromosome 13 leads to trisomy 13 syndrome or Patau's syndrome. Cases with trisomy 13 mosaicism most often show a less severe clinical phenotype. Survivors have severe mental retardation and fail to thrive [29]. Patients with trisomy 8 syndrome revealed mild to severe mental deficiency with craniofacial and skeletal abnormalities. Majority of patients are mosaic while full trisomy is lethal in embryonic stage [30].

Besides autosomes, sex chromosomes are also involved in different types of congenital disorders. In 45X (Turner syndrome), nondisjunction of paternal X chromosome is responsible for its origin [31]. Consistent clinical features include female in appearance with short stature, increased carrying angles at the elbows, broad chest with widely spaced nipples, and ovarian dysgenesis. In Klinefelter syndrome, chromosome analysis revealed 47XXY karyotype where patient is characterized by relatively tall stature, hypogonadism with small testes, and inadequate testosterone production. Virilization is partial with gynaecomastia [32]. On the other hand, hermaphroditism is not very frequent in occurrence where an individual has both male and female gonads. External genitalia is also ambiguous in nature. Most patients with true hermaphroditism have a 46XX karyotype with X chromosome, which derived from paternal source carries Y chromosome specific DNA sequences, originated as a result of crossing over. Surgical intervention in early childhood could repair the ambiguous external genitalia and provide either a male or female sex matching the karyotype of the respective individuals.

Deletion 5p syndrome is originated due to partial deletion of the short arm of the chromosome number 5 (5p-). This syndrome is also known as Cri Du Chat syndrome because there is a mewing cry or cat-like cry after birth due to abnormal laryngeal development, and in most cases the deleted chromosome is of paternal origin. There are multiple clinical abnormalities along with severe mental retardation and failure to thrive [33]. In duplication 15q syndrome there is a duplication of distal arm (q) of chromosome 15. Patients are characterized by growth deficiency, craniofacial abnormalities, and congenital heart defects [34].

Progress in the understanding of the etiology and pathogenesis of different congenital disorders and technological advancement in the identification of abnormal fetus before birth have made it possible the prenatal diagnosis of child having congenital abnormalities. There are several methods for prenatal diagnosis such as amniocentesis where chromosome analysis is made using amniotic fluid collected at 11–12 weeks of pregnancy [35]. On the other hand, noninvasive serum screening involves triple markers such as alpha feto protein, human chorionic gonadotropin, and unconjugated estriol [36]. Association of neural tube defect and high levels of alpha fetoprotein (AFP) in serum samples as well as in amniotic fluid are also important markers for prenatal diagnosis of chromosomal disorders [37]. Currently, screening techniques involving sequencing and genotyping of fetal DNA are most promising techniques for rapid prenatal diagnosis of chromosomal abnormalities [38]. The complex nature of Down syndrome and other chromosome abnormalities create the need for collaborative, multidisciplinary research to understand the complex pathophysiology of these syndromes.

Author details

Subrata Kumar Dey
Swami Vivekananda University, West Bengal, India

*Address all correspondence to: subratadey184@gmail.com

References

[1] Hassold T, Chen N, Funkhouser J, Joss T, Manuel B, et al. A cytogenetic study of 1000 spontaneous abortions. Annals of Human Genetics. 1980;**44**(2): 151-178

[2] Hassold TJ, Jacob PA. Trisomy in man. Annual Review of Genetics. 1984;**18**:69-97

[3] Nicolaidis P, Peterson MB. Origin and mechanism of nondisjunction in human autosomal trisomies. Human Reproduction. 1998;**13**:313-319

[4] Korenberg JR, Chen XN, Schipper R, Sun Z, Gonsky S, Carpenter N, et al. Down syndrome phenotypes: the consequences of chromosomal imbalance. Proceedings of the National Acadamy of Sciences USA. 1994;**91**: 4997-5001

[5] Mueller RF, Young ID. Emery's Elements of Genetics. 9th ed. UK: Churchill Livingstone; 1996. p. 215

[6] Antonarakis SE. Parental origin of the extra chromosome in trisomy 21 as indicated by analysis of DNA polymorphisms. The New England Journal of Medicine. 1991;**324**:872-876

[7] Peterson MB, Frantzen M, Antonarakis SE, Warren AC, Van Broeckhoven C, Chakravarti A, et al. Comparative study of microsatellite and cytogenetic markers for detecting the origin of the non disjoined chromosome 21 in Down syndrome. American Journal of Human Genetics. 1992;**51**:516-528

[8] Hassold T, Chiu D. Maternal age specific rates of numerical chromosome abnormalities with special reference to trisomy. Human Genetics. 1991;**70**:11-17

[9] Sherman SL, Takaesu N, Freeman SB, Grantham M, Phillips C, Blackston RD, et al. Trisomy 21: Association between reduced recombination and nondisjunction. American Journal of Human Genetics. 1991;**49**:608-620

[10] Ghosh S, Feingold E, Dey SK. Etiology of Down syndrome: Evidence for consistent association among altered meiotic recombination, nondisjunction and maternal age across populations. American Journal of Medical Genetics. 2009;**Part A 9999**:1-6

[11] Niebuhr E. Down syndrome: The possibility of a pathogenic segment on chromosome no. 21. Humangenetic. 1974;**2**:99-101

[12] Patterson D. The integrated map of human chromosome 21. In: Etiology and pathogenesis of down syndrome. Vol. 1. New York: Wiley-Liss; 1995. pp. 43-45

[13] Gardiner K, Slavov D, Bechtel L, Davisson M. Annotation of human chromosome 21 for relevance to Down syndrome: Gene structure and expression analysis. Genomics. 2002;**79**:833-843

[14] Ghosh S, Hong CS, Feigngold E, Ghosh P, Bhaumik P, Dey SK. Epidemiology of down syndrome: New insight into the multidimensional interactions among genetic and environmental risk factors in oocytes. American Journal of Epidemiology. 2011;**174**(9):1009-1016. DOI: 10.1093/aje/Kwn240

[15] Yang Q, Sherman SL, Hassold TJ, Allran K, Taft L, Pettay D, et al. Risk factors for trisomy 21 maternal cigarette smoking and oral contraceptive use in a population based case-control study. Genetics in Medicine. 1999;**1**:80-88

[16] Henderson J, Kesmodel U, Gray R. Systematic review of the fetal effects of prenatal binge-drinking. Journal of

Epidemiology and Community Health. 2007;**61**:1069-1073

[17] Allen EG, Freeman SB, Druschel C, Hobbs CA, O'Leary LA, Romitti PA, et al. Maternal age and risk for trisomy 21 assessed by the origin of chromosome nondisjunction: A report from the Atlanta and National Down syndrome projects. Human Genetics. 2009;**125**:41-52

[18] Reeves RH, Irving NG, Moran TH, Wohn A, Kitt C, Sisodia SS, et al. A mouse model for Down syndrome exhibits learning and behavioural deficits. Nature Genetics. 1995;**11**:177-184

[19] Sago H, Carlson EJ, Smith DJ, Rubin EM, Crinic LS, Huang TT, et al. Genetic dissection of region associated with behavioral abnormalities in mouse models for Down syndrome. Pediatric Research. 2000;**48**:606-613

[20] Gardiner K, Fortana A, Bechtel L, Davisson MT. Mouse models of Down syndrome: How useful can they be? Comparison of the gene content of human chromosome 21 with orthologous mouse genomic region. Gene. 2003;**318**:137-147

[21] Xing Z, Li Y, Pao A, Kaas G, Eugene Y. CRISPR/Cas9-facilitated chromosome engineering to model human chromosomal alterations. Advances in Research on Down Syndrome. 2017;**1**:108-113. DOI: 10.5772/intechopen.68260

[22] Freeman SB, Taft LF, Dooley KJ, Allran K, Sherman SL, Hassold TJ, et al. Population based study of congenital heart defects in Down syndrome. American Journal of Medical Genetics. 1998;**80**:213-217

[23] Ghosh P, Bhaumik P, Ghosh S, Ozbek U, Feingold E, Maslen C, et al. Polymorphic haplotype of CRELD1 differentially predispose Down syndrome and euploids individuals to atrioventricular septal defects. American Journal of Medical Genetics. 2012; **158A**(11):2843-2848. DOI: 10.1002/ajmg.a.35626

[24] Wilcock DM, Griffin WS. Down syndrome, neuroinflammation and Alzheimer's neuropathogenesis. Journal of Neuroinflammation. 2013;**10**:84-90

[25] Bhaumik P, Ghosh P, Biswas A, Ghosh S, Pal S, Sarkar B, et al. Rare intronic variations in TP73 gene found in patients with Alzheimer's Disease. International Journal of Human Genetics. 2017;**17**(4):158-168

[26] Kudo K. Myeloid leukemia associated with Down syndrome. Down Syndrome (Intech Publisher). 2013;7:108-113. DOI: 10.5772/52784

[27] Clift AK, Carol AC, Coupland CA, Keogh RH, Hemingway H, Hpppisley-Cox J. Mortality risk in Down syndrome: Results from a cohort study of 8 million adults. Annals of Internal Medicine. 2021;**174**:572-576. DOI: 10.7326/M20-4986/2021

[28] Edwards JH. A new trisomic syndrome. Lancet. 1960;**1**:787

[29] Patau K. Multiple congenital anomaly caused by an extra chromosome. Lancet. 1960;**1**:790

[30] Stadler GR, Buhler EM, Weber JR. Possible trisomy in chromosome group. Lancet. 1963;**1**(1379):6-12

[31] Turner HH. A syndrome of infantilism, congenital webbed neck and cubitus valgus. Endocrinology. 1938;**23**:566

[32] Klinefelter HF Jr, Reifenstein EC Jr, Albright F. Syndrome characterized by gynecomastia, a spermatogenesis without aleydigism and increased secretion of follicle stimulating hormone (gyn ecomastia). The Journal of Clinical Endocrinology and Metabolism. 1942;**2**:615

[33] Lejeune J. Trios cas de deletion partielle du bras court du chromosome 5. C R Acad Sci (D)(Paris). 1963; **257**:3098

[34] Fujimoto A. Inherited partial duplication of chromosome no. 15. Journal of Medical Genetics. 1974;**11**:287

[35] Golbus MS, Loughman WD, Epstein CJ. Prenatal genetic diagnosis in 3000 amniocenteses. The New England Journal of Medicine. 1979;**300**:157

[36] Bogart MH, Pandian MR, Jones OW. Abnormal maternal serum chorionic gonadotropin levels in pregnancies with fetal chromosome abnormalities. Prenatal Diagnosis. 1987;7:623-630

[37] Brock DJ, Sutcliffee RG. Alpha fetoprotein in the antenatal diagnosis of anencephaly and spina bifida. Lancet. 1972;**29**(7770):197-199

[38] Chiu RW, Chan KC, Gao Y, Lau VY, Zheng W, Leung TY. Non invasive prenatal diagnosis of fetal chromosomal aneuploidy by massively parallel genomic sequencing of DNA in maternal plasma. Proceedings National Acadamy of Sciences USA. 2008;**105**:20458-20463

Section 2

Mechanisms of Aneuploidy and Role of Polyploidy in Evolution

Chapter 2

Mechanisms of Aneuploidy

Emine Ikbal Atli

Abstract

Aneuploidy is a very common occurrence in humans and occurs in an estimated 20–40% of all pregnancies. It is the most prominent cause of miscarriages and congenital defects in humans and is the main obstacle to infertility treatment. The vast majority of aneuploidies are caused by maternal meiotic non-disjunction errors. High levels of recombination errors were observed in studies on fetal oocytes. This suggests that some oocytes are more prone to not being separated due to events occurring before birth. Cell cycle checkpoints that work in the meiotic phase and metaphase-anaphase transition work more moderately in women than in men. As a result, while there are abnormal cells that have been sorted out in spermatogenesis, in females these cells can escape the actual control and ultimately give rise to aneuploid eggs.

Keywords: nondisjunction, abnormal segregation, chromosome

1. Introduction

Although aneuploidy is a serious health problem, the reasons behind this phenomenon have not been fully confirmed. The development of a comprehensive set of tests is necessary for the evaluation and detection of aneugenic chemicals. The reliability of any aneuploidy analysis is always questioned by the fact that the mechanisms that cause aneuploidy are poorly understood, in part due to the multitude of factors involved in the occurrence of chromosome segregation and nondisjunction [1]. Errors in chromosome segregation during meiosis are usually seen in human oocytes and cause aneuploidy in embryos. These errors increase dramatically in the eggs of older women.

Here, we attempt to summarize recent studies commenting on how progressive disruption of chromosome structures contributes to age-related aneuploidy. In addition, various cellular pathways that cause aneuploidy in oocytes of women of all ages are being investigated. Data from mouse and human oocytes are discussed with emphasis on studies focusing on this phenomenon in humans [2].

2. Meiosis in human oocytes

Meiosis involves two sequential cell divisions in which homologous chromosomes (meiosis I) are separated in the first stage, followed by sister chromatids (meiosis II). In the first meiosis, the homologous chromosomes separate from each other, then the homologous chromosomes are joined together. These connections are established early in oocyte development during the growth of the female fetus in a process called homologous recombination. The maternal and paternal chromosomes are first compressed by the synaptonemal complex and then crossed over. After crossover, new sister chromatids are formed, containing adjacent portions of maternal and paternal sister chromatids. Cohesin complexes that previously linked sister chromatids of each homologous chromosome now link homologous chromosomes together: Cohesin (distal cohesin) distal to the crossover sites connects homologs, while cohesin (proximal cohesin) between crossover sites and centromeres continues to bind sister chromatids [3]. The chromosome configuration that turns out to be two homologous chromosomes is called bivalent. As meiosis I occurs, the bivalents must be oriented on the spindle so that the two sister chromatids contained in each homologous chromosome face the same spindle pole. The kinetochores of sister chromatids must behave as a single kinetochore. It is thought that adding sister kinetochores to a functional location will facilitate this function. Oocytes then enter a state of cellular stagnation called 'interphase' in processes spanning different periods of time. The functional units of oocyte and somatic cells in the ovary are called follicles [4–6]. During storage, the oocytes remain small and are surrounded by a single layer of squamous cell epithelium called the "primordial follicle". Periodically, some primordial follicles begin to grow. Somatic cells supply the oocyte with macromolecular precursors through gap junctions, and oocyte volume increases significantly. This enrichment of nutrients prepares the oocyte [7, 8] to mature into an egg, which after fertilization can give rise to an embryo.

Oocytes emerge from dictyate arrest after puberty. In the middle of the menstrual cycle, the rise of luteinizing hormone from the pituitary gland causes the oocyte to continue meiosis and mature into a fertilizable egg. First, the nucleus disintegrates and sets of meiotic spindles are formed, which align the chromosomes in meiosis I metaphase. The spindle progresses to the oocyte cortex, where homologous chromosomes separate. One set of homologous chromosomes remains in the oocyte, while the other is extruded into the first polar body formed. Molecularly, the segregation of chromosomes during meiosis I is activated by the cleavage of Rec8, a meiosis-specific subunit of the cohesin complex [9]. Rec8 is cleaved by Separase, which is activated along with anaphase. During anaphase I, only the cohesin in the arm region is broken down so that the chromosomes can separate from each other. Cohesin in the centromeric regions is protected from cleavage by Shugoshin proteins (Sgo), so that sister chromatids stay together during anaphase I. As meiosis II occurs, the second meiotic spindle fuses [10–13]. The maturing egg has transitioned to the quiescent phase in metaphase II and is transported to the fallopian tube during ovulation. The egg waits to complete its second meiosis until it is fertilized by the sperm. As the second meiosis continues, the Sgo proteins migrate to the kinetochores, and in anaphase II, the cleavage of the centromeric cohesin takes place [14–17]. In order to complete meiosis, the sister chromatids of the remaining chromosomes, the oocyte and the second polar body, must be formed. Chromosomes from the oocyte and sperm separate as the pronuclear envelope and then stand ready for the first mitotic division of the embryo. The embryo then divides into a multicellular blastocyst and implants in the uterus to develop further [18–20].

3. Types of aneuploidy in oocytes

Recent technological advances have increased the chances of catching aneuploidy in eggs or in the early stages of embryonic development. In pre-implantation genetic diagnosis, an embryo may sometimes be biopsied and analyzed for genetic abnormalities to select healthy embryos for implantation. As an alternative to this technique, testing oocytes can minimize the need to test embryos. In particular, polar bodies can be used to determine the cytology of an oocyte without damaging it [21, 22]. The use of polar bodies for aneuploidy detection in IVF applications also facilitates embryo selection before implantation [23, 24]. Genetic analysis of both polar bodies can accurately detect aneuploidy in mature oocyte because all chromosomal copies are extruded into polar bodies [25–27]. For example, an excess chromosome in the first polar body indicates loss of the homolog of that chromosome in the oocyte after meiosis I, while an incorrect chromosome number in the second polar body indicates a chromosome segregation error in meiosis II. On the other hand, the second polar body is formed only after fertilization. Chromosomes from biopsied polar bodies are best previously analyzed by fluorescent in situ hybridization (FISH). Although widely used for embryo selection, clinical applications of FISH are only informative for a particular chromosome and results may be inaccurate [28]. New, more sensitive methods such as Sequence Comparative Genome Hybridization (aCGH) and next-generation sequencing (NGS) platforms provide improved statistics for aneuploidy prevalence and better characterization of segregation errors [29].

Two classical ways that have been suggested to account for chromosome segregation errors in meiosis are nondisjunction (NDJ) and premature separation of sister chromatids (PSSC). For NDJ, homologous chromosomes or sister chromatids cannot separate at meiosis I or meiosis II, respectively. Similar segregation errors are seen between meiosis I and II, although meiosis II error rates have sometimes been reported to be higher.

This can be explained by the fact that errors that can be seen in meiosis I occur in meiosis II, because early cleavage sister chromatids can separate correctly in meiosis I, while errors are observed later in meiosis II.

Surprisingly, PSSC mutations in meiosis I could be corrected by a 'balance' error during meiosis II: if both the first and second polar bodies share mutual errors (for example, a loss in the polar body first followed by a second gain in the polar body; or vice versa) the resulting oocyte will have the correct number of chromosomes [30, 31].

Chromosome pairs 15, 16, 21, and 22 are the chromosomes that most commonly contribute to human aneuploidies, but data on the contributions of other chromosomes are lacking due to limited statistical information for types of aneuploidy. Frequently, an oocyte will experience simultaneous errors involving more than one chromosome, suggesting that some oocytes are susceptible to global dysfunction. This effect is also evident in embryos where up to 42% of detected aneuploidies contain more than one chromosome [32, 33].

However, the etiology of embryonic aneuploidy is more complex, as errors can also occur from sperm or during rapid mitotic divisions in embryogenesis [34, 35]. Advances in single-cell whole genome amplification (WGA) allow unprecedented characterization of genomic content within polar bodies.

Analyzes of the genomes of polar body-oocyte and polar body-embryo triplets (i.e. a biopsy of an oocyte or embryo fused with first and second polar bodies) revealed an alternative mechanism of segregation, termed 'reverse segregation' [36].

Reverse segregation occurs when sister chromatids separate at meiosis I so that there are no homologous chromosomes.

Reverse segregation results in the correct number of chromosome cells. The chromatid pairs, the copies inherited by the oocyte and first pole body, have different parental origins and are heterozygous at the centromeres.

After meiosis I, their connection is broken and during metaphase II, alignment problems may occur in the spindle fibers. In one study; although it was the most observed error in number, reverse segregation was detected in less than 10% of the triples analyzed [36]. Interestingly, all of the donors participating in this study produced at least one oocyte or embryo that underwent reverse segregation.

The oocytes included in this study were obtained from women aged 33–41 years. A similar study examining oocytes from younger donors aged 25–35 years reported that no reverse segregation was observed [26, 36].

4. Causes of aneuploidy increasing with age

Women experience a gradual decrease in their ability to get pregnant as they age. Loss of reproductive ability usually occurs approximately 10 years after the age of 35. Meiotic chromosome segregation errors increase very clearly in women of this age group. A large-scale cytogenetic analysis examining more than 20,000 human oocytes by FISH reported that aneuploidy occurred in 20% of oocytes retrieved from women aged 35 years, increasing to approximately 60% in women over 43 years of age [37].

Current studies with aCGH have confirmed that the rates of aneuploidy increase dramatically in oocytes from older women [23, 27, 38–40]. Conservation of bivalents is crucial for correct chromosome segregation. However, recent studies in human oocytes reveal that the structure of bivalents is prone to fragmentation in oocytes of older women.

In mice and humans, two major structural defects occur with increasing age in bivalents. First, sister kinetochores disperse over long distances, which is incompatible and often associated with incorrect attachment to the meiotic spindle. Second, the bivalents formed in senescent oocytes are more often separated into individual chromosomes, called univalents. Univalent pairs may split uncoordinatedly and may also contribute to aneuploidy. Interestingly, it is possible for both defects to result in an inverse decomposition pattern, as we will discuss below [41–44].

Sister chromatids in mouse and human oocytes lose compatibility with age, which can cause misalignment of bivalents in meiosis I.

Loosely related sister chromatids may no longer function properly as they align on the meiotic spindle. In human oocytes, separated sister kinetochores tend to form more merotelic attachment to spindle microtubules.

In addition, other age-related factors may promote defective kinetochore-microtubule attachments.

Excessive segregation of sister kinetochores in human oocytes causes bivalents to take on unexpected alignments in the meiotic spindle. In a newly defined bivalent configuration called 'inverted bivalents', the bivalents are rotated to the spindle axis: the sister chromatids of a homologous chromosome misalign and misalign, linking microtubules at opposite spindle poles instead of orienting them to the same spindle pole, as in mitosis [45–48].

Both half and fully inverted bivalents occur. Only one pair of sister chromatids is attached to opposite spindle poles in semi-inverted bivalents, while both pairs are attached to opposite poles in fully inverted bivalents. Reverse bivalents have been observed more frequently in oocytes from older females and are associated with increasing distances between sister kinetochores. Since sister chromatids are oriented separately on the spindle, similar to mitosis, fully inverted bivalents can lead to an inverse pattern of segregation. Bivalents also sometimes appear bent along their axis because homologous chromosomes rotate relative to each other, which can put more pressure on the already weakened cohesion.

The age-related loss of balance applicable to bivalents is not limited to the pericentromeric regions surrounding the kinetochores. There is also danger in the harmony that connects homologous chromosomes. Homologous chromosome pairs in bivalents often remain separated by large gaps in oocytes of aged mouse and human females. These and similar structural defects are indicative of decreased compatibility between bivalent homologous chromosomes. In more complex cases, bivalents sometimes divide earlier into two separate chromosomes (univalents) before anaphase I. The prevalence of univalents increases exponentially with age, occurring in 40% of oocytes in women older than 35 years and 10% of oocytes in women aged 30–35 years. In mouse oocytes, univalent alignment problems can cause chromosome separation errors. Univalents in mouse and human oocytes could also align on the first meiotic spindle, similar to mitotic chromosomes, with both sister kinetochores facing opposite spindle poles. This can create a mitosis-like pattern of segregation and result in reverse segregation: equal segregation of both univalents into sister chromatids will result in the correct chromosome number acquired by the oocyte and the first polar body, but the chromatids will originate from different parental origins. However, the sister chromatids have been divided much earlier and could not be properly aligned to the spindle at metaphase II.

The molecular mechanisms that may cause these dramatic developments in chromosomal organization in human oocytes, which change with advancing age, are still unresolved. However, studies in mice have clarified the loss of cohesin as a major contributor to age-related aneuploidy. Cohesin complexes containing Rec8 in mouse oocytes are already present during DNA replication in the early stages of meiosis. After fertilization, they are thought to be renewed when DNA is replicated again in the embryo. Therefore, the cohesin complexes must remain in place during the prolonged period of dictation arrest to ensure correct chromosome segregation in meiosis. Rec8 levels are severely reduced in bivalents of oocytes from naturally aged mice [48–51].

5. Conclusions

Fertility declines gradually as women age, and by midlife women begin to lose their ability to produce healthy eggs. Meiotic chromosomes experience increased age-related structural changes that can result in increased Error rates in chromosome segregation. Newly described processes have been identified in human oocyte structures that may explain the emergence of an alternative form of segregation. Conducted studies will better reveal why oocytes are often defective, leading to age-related infertility. Recent studies have reported that meiosis in mammalian females is inherently error-prone, leading to high aneuploidy and sterility. The cellular pathways responsible for chromosome separations are prone to error and affect females of all ages.

Acknowledgements

I would like to thank my supervisors Hakan Gurkan for all his help and advice.

Conflict of interest

The authors declare no conflict of interest.

Acronyms and abbreviations

IVF	in-vitro fertilization
FISH	fluorescent in situ hybridization

a CGH array Comparative Genome Hybridization
NDJ nondisjunction
PSSC premature separation of sister chromatids
WGA whole genome amplification

Author details

Emine Ikbal Atli
Trakya University Faculty of Medicine, Department of Medical Genetics, Turkey Balkan Campus, Edirne, Turkey

*Address all correspondence to: emine.ikbal@gmail.com; eikbalatli@trakya.edu.tr

References

[1] Seoane AI, Güerci AM, Dulout FN. Mechanisms involved in the induction of aneuploidy: The significance of chromosome loss. Genetics and Molecular Biology. 2000, 2000;**23**(4): 1077-1082

[2] Webster A, Schuh M. Mechanisms of Aneuploidy in Human Eggs. Trends Cell Biol. 2017;**27**(1):55-68

[3] Sakuno T, Watanabe Y. Studies of meiosis disclose distinct roles of cohesion in the core centromere and pericentromeric regions. Chromosome Research. 2009;**17**:239-249

[4] Toth A et al. Functional genomics identifies monopolin: A kinetochore protein required for segregation of homologs during meiosis i. Cell. 2000;**103**:1155-1168

[5] Rabitsch KP et al. Kinetochore recruitment of two nucleolar proteins is required for homolog segregation in meiosis I. Developmental Cell. 2003;**4**: 535-548

[6] Yokobayashi S, Watanabe Y. The kinetochore protein Moa1 enables cohesion-mediated monopolar attachment at meiosis I. Cell. 2005;**123**: 803-817

[7] Peters H. The development of the mouse ovary from birth to maturity. Acta Endocrinologica. 1969;**62**:98-116

[8] Herlands RL, Schultz RM. Regulation of Mouse oocyte growth: probable nutritional role for intercellular communication between follicle cells and oocytes in oocyte growth. The Journal of Experimental Zoology. 1984;**229**:317-325

[9] Watanabe Y, Nurse P. Cohesin Rec8 is required for reductional chromosome segregation at meiosis. Nature. 1999; **400**:461-464

[10] Buonomo SB et al. Disjunction of homologous chromosomes in meiosis I depends on proteolytic cleavage of the meiotic cohesin Rec8 by separin. Cell. 2000;**103**:387-398

[11] Llano E et al. Shugoshin-2 is essential for the completion of meiosis but not for mitotic cell division in mice. Genes & Development. 2008;**22**: 2400-2413

[12] Lee J et al. Unified mode of centromeric protection by shugoshin in mammalian oocytes and somatic cells. Nature Cell Biology. 2008;**10**:42-52

[13] Gomez R et al. Mammalian SGO2 appears at the inner centromere domain and redistributes depending on tension across centromeres during meiosis II and mitosis. EMBO Reports. 2007;**8**: 173-180

[14] Lee J et al. Unified mode of centromeric protection by shugoshin in mammalian oocytes and somatic cells. Nature Cell Biology. 2008;**10**:42-52

[15] Gomez R et al. Mammalian SGO2 appears at the inner centromere domain and redistributes depending on tension across centromeres during meiosis II and mitosis. EMBO Reports. 2007;**8**:173-180

[16] Clift D, Schuh M. Restarting life: Fertilization and the transition from meiosis to mitosis. Nature Reviews. Molecular Cell Biology. 2013;**14**: 549-562

[17] Chambon JP et al. The PP2A inhibitor I2PP2A is essential for sister chromatid segregation in oocyte meiosis II. Current Biology. 2013;**23**:485-490

[18] Clift D, Schuh M. Restarting life: fertilization and the transition from meiosis to mitosis. Nature Reviews. Molecular Cell Biology. 2013;**14**:549-562

[19] Chambon JP et al. The PP2A inhibitor I2PP2A is essential for sister chromatid segregation in oocyte meiosis II. Current Biology. 2013;**23**:485-490

[20] Courtois A et al. The transition from meiotic to mitotic spindle assembly is gradual during early mammalian development. The Journal of Cell Biology. 2012;**198**:357-370

[21] Brezina PR et al. Preimplantation genetic testing for aneuploidy: What technology should you use and what are the differences? Journal of Assisted Reproduction and Genetics. 2016;**33**: 823-832

[22] Montag M et al. Polar body biopsy: A viable alternative to preimplantation genetic diagnosis and screening. Reproductive Biomedicine Online. 2009;**18**(Suppl. 1):6-11

[23] Geraedts J et al. Polar body array CGH for prediction of the status of the corresponding oocyte Part I: clinical results. Human Reproduction. 2011;**26**: 3173-3180

[24] Magli MC et al. Polar body array CGH for prediction of the status of the corresponding oocyte Part II: technical aspects. Human Reproduction. 2011;**26**: 3181-3185

[25] Verlinsky Y et al. Analysis of the first polar body: preconception genetic diagnosis. Human Reproduction. 1990;**5**:826-829

[26] Hou Y et al. Genome analyses of single human oocytes. Cell. 2013;**155**: 1492-1506

[27] Handyside AH et al. Multiple meiotic errors caused by predivision of chromatids in women of advanced maternal age undergoing in vitro fertilisation. European Journal of Human Genetics. 2012;**20**:742-747

[28] Harper J et al. What next for preimplantation genetic screening (PGS)? A position statement from the ESHRE PGD Consortium Steering Committee. Human Reproduction. 2010;**25**:821-823

[29] Fragouli E et al. Cytogenetic analysis of human blastocysts with the use of FISH, CGH and aCGH: Scientific data and technical evaluation. Human Reproduction. 2011;**26**:480-490

[30] Treff NR et al. Next generation sequencing-based comprehensive chromosome screening in mouse polar bodies, oocytes, and embryos. Biology of Reproduction. 2016;**94**:76

[31] Fragouli E et al. The cytogenetics of polar bodies: insights into female meiosis and the diagnosis of aneuploidy. Molecular Human Reproduction. 2011;**17**:286-295

[32] Sills ES et al. Determining parental origin of embryo aneuploidy: analysis of genetic error observed in 305 embryos derived from anonymous donor oocyte IVF cycles. Molecular Cytogenetics. 2014;**7**:68

[33] Templado C et al. Aneuploidy in human spermatozoa. Cytogenetic and Genome Research. 2011;**133**:91-99

[34] Pacchierotti F et al. Gender effects on the incidence of aneuploidy in mammalian germ cells. Environmental Research. 2007;**104**:46-69

[35] Chow JF et al. Array comparative genomic hybridization analyses of all blastomeres of a cohort of embryos from young IVF patients revealed significant contribution of mitotic errors to embryo mosaicism at the cleavage stage. Reproductive Biology and Endocrinology. 2014;**12**:105

[36] Ottolini CS et al. Genome-wide maps of recombination and chromosome segregation in human oocytes and embryos show selection for

maternal recombination rates. Nature Genetics. 2015;**47**:727-735

[37] Kuliev A et al. Meiosis errors in over 20,000 oocytes studied in the practice of preimplantation aneuploidy testing. Reproductive Biomedicine Online. 2011;**22**:2-8

[38] Feichtinger M et al. Increasing live birth rate by pre- implantation genetic screening of pooled polar bodies using array comparative genomic hybridization. PLoS One. 2015;**10**:e0128317

[39] Gabriel AS et al. Array comparative genomic hybridisation on first polar bodies suggests that non-disjunction is not the predominant mechanism leading to aneuploidy in humans. Journal of Medical Genetics. 2011;**48**: 433-437

[40] Fragouli E et al. The cytogenetics of polar bodies: insights into female meiosis and the diagnosis of aneuploidy. Molecular Human Reproduction. 2011;**17**:286-295

[41] Duncan FE et al. Chromosome cohesion decreases in human eggs with advanced maternal age. Aging Cell. 2012;**11**:1121-1124

[42] Zielinska AP et al. Sister kinetochore splitting and precocious disintegration of bivalents could explain the maternal age effect. eLife. 2015;**4**:e11389

[43] Patel J et al. Unique geometry of sister kinetochores in human oocytes during meiosis I may explain maternal age-associated increases in chromosomal abnormalities. Biology Open. 2015;**5**: 178-184

[44] Sakakibara Y et al. Bivalent separation into univalents precedes age-related meiosis I errors in oocytes. Nature Communications. 2015;**6**:7550

[45] Zielinska AP et al. Sister kinetochore splitting and precocious disintegration of bivalents could explain the maternal age effect. eLife. 2015;**4**:e11389

[46] Shomper M et al. Kinetochore microtubule establishment is defective in oocytes from aged mice. Cell Cycle. 2014;**13**:1171-1179

[47] Patel J et al. Unique geometry of sister kinetochores in human oocytes during meiosis I may explain maternal age-associated increases in chromosomal abnormalities. Biology Open. 2015;**5**: 178-184

[48] Sakakibara Y et al. Bivalent separation into univalents precedes age-related meiosis I errors in oocytes. Nature Communications. 2015;**6**:7550

[49] Lister LM et al. Age-related meiotic segregation errors in mammalian oocytes are preceded by depletion of cohesin and Sgo2. Current Biology. 2010;**20**:1511-1521

[50] Hunt P et al. Analysis of chromosome behavior in intact mammalian oocytes: Monitoring the segregation of a univalent chromosome during female meiosis. Human Molecular Genetics. 1995;**4**:2007-2012

[51] Nagaoka SI et al. Oocyte-specific differences in cellcycle control create an innate susceptibility to meiotic errors. Current Biology. 2011;**21**:651-657

Chapter 3

The Unique Existence of Chromosomal Abnormalities in Polyploidy Plants

Van Hieu Pham

Abstract

Chromosomal abnormalities are a popular natural phenomenon, especially in polyploid plants, and their unique existence in plants is one of the major forces for speciation and evolution. This means that plants with existing chromosomal abnormalities developing through sexual and asexual pathways shed light on increasing biomass and adapting ecology. Regarding the former, plants with chromosomal abnormalities experience not only enlargement effects but also increased phytochemical compounds. As far as ecological perspectives are concerned, chromosomal abnormalities in plants enhance biotic and abiotic tolerance to climate change. This chapter focuses on chromosomal abnormalities in whole genome doubling, such as autopolyploid, allopolyploid, and aneuploidy plants, and discusses the effects and benefits of these abnormalities to evolution and ecological adaptation at the individual and population levels. It also discusses some advantages and disadvantages of polyploid animals in comparison with polyploid plants.

Keywords: chromosomal abnormality, polyploidy, evolution, climate change, reproduction

1. Introduction

Darwin's theory of natural selection maintains that the polymorphism that exhibits gross chromosomal alteration in plants as a way to reciprocally translocate along with changes in the segregation of pairs of chromosomes to ensure heterozygosity maintenance and limitation of the expression of lethal genes. Every day, living organisms ingest all kinds of food, taking in energy and nutrients to nourish, maintain, and develop their bodies. As such, food security is vitally important to survival. Attaining food security, however, has been a challenge. Potential solutions to food insecurity might lie in the genetic mechanisms regulating the reproductive process of plants. Different organisms reproduce in different ways, either via sexual combining of male and female gametes or asexually. Asexual reproduction generates a new plant by using parts of the parent plants. Some artificial asexual reproduction methods include grafting, layering, and micropropagation. Genetic identicalness to the progenitor plant is an outstanding feature of plants produced asexually. Reproductive chromosome abnormalities derive from mistaking meiosis and mitosis occur [1]. For instance, observing meiotic processes revealed evidence that the trio of genes *SMG7*, *SDS*, and *MS5* interrelated with both other chromatin organizing factors and proteins functioning DNA repair-related, involved in *MSH6* and *DAYSLEEPER*. The convergent tasks detected (other meiotic pathways, chromosome arrangement or remodeling, ABA cues and ion transport) offer insights into the challenges of polyploidization. Investigation of the meiosis of autotetraploid potato *Solanum tuberosum* revealed a variety of challenges in correct segregation and recombination of multiple homologous chromosomes that constrain meiotic chromosomal configuration [2].

With advances in genetic engineering and continual elucidation of genes governing the reproductive pathway, humanity is on the verge of being able to control the expression and regulation of these genes [1, 3]. Key genes related to flowering, such as *CO*, *CRY2*, *FT*, *FPF1*, *FD*, *GA1*, and *ELA1*, have already been studied [3]. Scientists and breeders worldwide use biotechnology to study reproductive processes in laboratories and field trials. Sustainable agricultural development is required to increase crop diversity, stabilize yield, and increase resilience via the accelerated development of several crops containing desired traits that have the capacity to adapt to and mitigate consequences from climate change [4, 5].

In terms of biodiversity, speciation, and evolution, there are thousands of existing plant species that can adapt to various topographies and climates. This means that plant species not only increase the abundance of genetics but also enhance the ability to adapt to boost genome evolution in harsh environments [1, 6]. The best examples are those that involve autopolyploids, allopolyploids, and aneuploidy. There are more than 4000 potato varieties, including more than 180 wild potato relatives [7]. More specifically, potato, one of the most multifaceted genetic modes with a variety of ploidy levels, such as 76%, recognizes diploids, 3% triploids, 12% tetraploids, 2% pentaploids, and 7% hexaploids, among which the highest yield is tetraploid due to a further level of genetic heterogeneity [8–10]. Based on practical empirical proof, two clusters of cultivated potato have been categorized: the Andigenum group located in the high Andes of northern and central South America that exhibit a wide range of ploidy levels, and the Chilotanum group from the lowlands of southern Chile, which are tetraploids [11].

Plant karyotypes at individual, species, and genera levels exhibit an abnormal number of chromosomes. A typical example is Chayote (*Saccharum edule* (Jacq.) Sw.) with variable chromosome numbers of 12, 13, and 14 resulting from cytological analysis [12], as shown in **Table 1**.

This chapter focuses on chromosomal abnormalities in whole genome doubling, such as autopolyploid, allopolyploid, and aneuploidy plants, and then discusses the effects and benefits of these abnormalities to evolution and ecological adaptation at the individual and population levels. It also discusses some advantages and disadvantages of polyploid animals in comparison with polyploid plants.

Species	n	2n	Source
Saccharum edule	11, 12, 13, 14	22, 24, 26, 28	[13–17]
Curcuma parviflora Wall.	14, 14, 16	28, 30, 32	[18]
Curcuma zedoaria Rosc.	21	63, 64	[19–23]
Curcuma longa L.	21	62, 63, 64	[19–22, 24]
Paspalum aff. arundinellum Mez	10	50, 51	[25]
Jacobaea vulgaris	20	30, 31	[26]
Brassica rapa L. ssp. *pekinensis*	10	20, 24	[27]

Table 1.
Summary of plant species with chromosomal abnormalities.

2. Chromosomal abnormalities affect giant effects and alternative natural secondary metabolites

That chromosomal abnormality outranks other plants in terms of parts of plant size and biochemical compounds characteristically states that gene regulation plays an important role. Regarding the upregulation of genes, cell division and cell expansion are related to genes such as ARGOS, *ANT* (*AITEGUMENTA*), *CYCD3;1*, *Growth Regulating Factor 1* (*AtGRF1*) and *EXPASIN 10* (*AtEXPA10*) [27–29], *EXPB3*, and *TCP* [30]. Alongside these genes, lipid transport genes such as *wbc11–2* and *cer5–2* are a way to make large autotetraploid plants [31–33]. Moreover, proteins involved in cell proliferation, glutathione metabolic pathways, and cellulose, chlorophyll, pectin, and lignin synthesis play a role in enlarging plant size [34, 35]. Cytosine methylation in the whole genome also contributes to changes in organ size in polyploid plants, which can effectively improve potential and complex agronomic traits in many crops [36, 37]. Cell size in polyploid plants plays an important role in changing phenotypes [38]. Enlarged organ size due to chromosomal abnormalities usually leads to increased yield and production of cultivated plants [39]. Studying autotetraploid *Vicia cracca* L. revealed that seed size and germination of tetraploids are more dominant than diploid seeds [40]. Although chromosomal abnormalities lead to large plants, autotetraploid birch plants (*Betula platyphylla*) and apple plants (*Malus domestica*) have a dwarf phenotype caused by reduced growth regulation signals [41, 42].

Similarly, chromosomal abnormalities also alter secondary metabolites, especially phytochemical compounds, in several plant species [43]. For example, natural components observed in tetrasomic tetraploid opium poppy (*Papaver somniferum* L.) enhanced morphine content by 25–50% by changing the expression of several genes regulating the alkaloid biosynthesis pathway [44]. Another example is cytosine methylation occurring genome-wide, enhancing phytochemicals in autotetraploid cymbopogons [36]. The autotetraploid *Arabidopsis thaliana* Col-0 alters metabolites and genes regulating tricarboxylic acid cycle (TCA) and gamma-Aminobutyric acid (GABA) compared with diploids [45]. Lycopene significantly increased autotriploid watermelons because of a regulation of phytohormones on metabolic pathways and upregulation of genes controlling biosynthetic lycopene [46]. Interestingly, polyploidization is a promising approach for gaining significant value, especially with medicinal plants, by producing secondary metabolites [43]. For example, upregulating genes contributing to the biosynthesis pathway of podophyllotoxin (PTOX) in autotetraploid *Linum album* enhanced the content of PTOX [47]. Vitamin A enrichment in triploid banana has been initiated by inducing tetraploids from several types of diploids and then creating hybrids [48]. Many total flavonoids and gastrodin are produced in autotetraploid *Anoectochilus formosanus* Hayata [49]. The tetraploid type of *Physalis angutala* Linn. from Rajasthan alters palmitic acid, linoleic acid, and linolenic acid [50]. In the last decade, many plant studies have given objects based on the outstanding benefits of chromosomal abnormalities. Those breeders have been observing chromosomal abnormalities as a way to gain elite plant cultivars because an increase in plant organ size is derived from some of the most significant consequences of chromosomal abnormalities [51, 52].

The chromosomal abnormality of the level of ploidy variation is useful for breeding both within and among autopolyploid and allopolyploid plant species [25]. Another view is that chromosomal abnormalities contribute to plants' ability to withstand detrimental environmental conditions. As far as the first idea is concerned, a chromosomal abnormality is not appropriate for sexual reproduction in aneuploidy due to chromosomal abnormalities in gametes. Another utilization of polyploidy is that grafted crops can use artificial polyploidy as parts of rootstock and scion with potential agronomic traits in the context of climate variability [53].

3. Chromosomal abnormalities enhance abiotic and biotic stress tolerance

Chromosomal abnormalities in plants enhance both biotic and abiotic stress tolerance. For example, many studies have proven that several pathways respond to salinity stress. Chromosomally abnormal flora use several processes to adapt to high salt concentration conditions, including accumulating Na+ extrusion in roots, increasing Na+ transport to leaves, regulating osmotics, enhancing gene expression related to antioxidants, mitigating reactive oxygen species (ROS), photosynthesizing cues, changing SNP markers related to salt stress, upregulating aquaporin genes, phytohormone transduction cues, protein processing, regulating transcription factors, upregulating ATP synthase to enhance ion transport and changing protons, and using miRNAs [54–63]. Chromosomally abnormal plants can also adapt to water insufficiency through miRNA mechanisms and target genes controlling transcriptional regulation, hormone metabolism, and plant defense. An increase in abscisic acid (ABA) content in response to drought stress in several polyploid plants such as *Paulownia fortunei*, *P. australis*, *P. tomentosa*, and *Lycium ruthenicum* has been observed [64–69]. Antioxidant defense systems were activated to sufficiently support heat tolerance in *Dioscorea* and *Arabidopsis* [70, 71]. Plants with chromosomal abnormalities might tolerate cold stress by growing antioxidants and epigenetics [72, 73]. Changing root anatomical characteristics supports autotetraploids to adapt to high concentrations of boron in soil and enhance Cu transport genes. Activation of antioxidation defense and positive regulation of ABA-responsive gene expression are ways to survive in environments containing high concentrations of copper [74, 75]. Enhancing the expression of target genes that regulate proline biosynthesis to support autopolyploid birch plants (*B. platyphylla*) in $NaHCO_3$ stress tolerance has been investigated [76]. In addition, biotic resistance was demonstrated in autotetraploid *Malus × domestica* and *Solanum chacoense*. More specifically, significantly increasing the *Rvi6* resistance gene locus was observed as a way to assist autopolyploids in enhancing *Venturia* resistance [77]. Similarly, autotetraploid potato has the capacity of common scab resistance by crossing 2n gametes from the diploid *S. chacoense* [78].

4. Chromosomal abnormalities help plants adapt to ecological invasion and climate variability

Chromosomal abnormalities are one of the major adaptation ecologies and climate changes, such as fixing on growth, potential morphological traits and ecological invasion, pollinators, and the factors supporting pollination in nature [79]. After appearance of chromosomal abnormality in some rare cases, the increasing cell size leads to alteration of physiological manners with their environmental condition, augmenting multiple novel alleles and changing regulatory pathways to create new potentially beneficial phenotypic variations. For instance, studying the transcriptome in aneuploidy maize revealed qualitative changes in gene expression in comparison to wild-type plants [80]. The number of expanding ecological spaces to polyploid plants has been recorded in various studies [81]. Polyploid *A. thaliana* is a plant with adaptive potential caused by the increased resources of transposable element (TE) insertions at higher ploidy levels and enhanced gene expression related to reproduction [82, 83]. Several studies have proven that chromosomal abnormalities adapt to ecological invasion and climate variation. For example, biological invasions in *Brassicaceae* proved to be evolutionary processes to adapt and widespread in central Europe [84]. Another example is that of the native range of distribution of *Lythrum salicaria*. Several cytotypes with 2×, 3×, 4×, and 6× variations are found in regions of the Middle East, while only tetraploids are located in North America. In addition, the invasive spread of North American populations lacks differences in ploidy level [85]. Studying potato germplasm demonstrated markers related to unique geographic identity associated with traits of abiotic stress tolerance [86]. One of the priorities in genotype development is to gain stress tolerance and beneficial nutritional aspects as a way to reduce the effects of climate change [87, 88]. The view is that polyploidization contributes to better adaptation to the environment in terms of suitability for growth and other benefits of cell size. Breeders and human beings can benefit immensely from more ecological adaptation after chromosomal abnormality since it improves potential traits being exploited for breeding experiments.

For the most part, polyploidy is probably less popular in the animal kingdom than in the plant kingdom. More specifically, polyploids have been observed in amphibia (African clawed frog, *Xenopus* spp.), and different species of fishes exist [89]. This is because the polyploid animal species can overcome meiosis and exhibit parthenogenesis in which an egg cell can develop into an individual without fertilization. In addition, polyploid animal kingdoms are similar to polyploid plant kingdoms. They both have beneficial and detrimental effects and are the reason for meiotic imbalance. The greatest advantage of polyploid animals is that polyploid offspring are shielded from the deleterious effects of recessive mutations. However, chromosomal abnormalities may lead to congenital diseases and pregnancy loss in animals, especially in humans. Regarding meiotic imbalance, spindle irregularities might occur in polyploids, resulting in chaotic segregation of chromatids and aneuploid cells. An abnormal number of chromosomes in aneuploid cells might result in three or more sets of chromosomes produced in meiosis being different from diploid cells. This can explain why polyploid animals could form multiple arrangements of homologous chromosomes in metaphase I, resulting in abnormal or random segregation to produce aneuploid gametes or to form imbalanced gametes [89, 90].

5. Conclusion

It is unquestionable whether chromosomal abnormalities derived from sex or asexual reproduction are essential for the successful existence of organisms on this planet. With climate variability becoming more alarming than ever, chromosomal abnormality has been occurring naturally as a way to address the issue of food security by expanding breeding opportunities to develop seedless triploid plants, increase ornamental features, increase environmental tolerance, enhance biomass, and more. Chromosomal abnormalities are also vital to human beings mainly because their exploration can open opportunities for securing food security. For example, breeders who are experienced in hybrid development are more likely to find desired agronomic traits. More importantly, several breeders today require at least a desired trait of novel crops before considering using them for production. Chromosomal abnormalities are essential for success in adapting ecology and play a vital role in evolution due to generating variation in a natural population.

Acknowledgements

The author thanks the financial support and convenient conditions from HCMC Biotechnology Center.

Author details

Van Hieu Pham
Biotechnology Center of Ho Chi Minh, Ho Chi Minh City, Vietnam

*Address all correspondence to: hieupvbio@gmail.com

References

[1] Bohutinska M, Alston M, Monnahan P, Mandakova T, Bray S, Paajanen P, et al. Novelty and convergence in adaptation to whole genome duplication. Molecular Biology and Evolution. 2021. DOI: 10.1093/molbev/msab096

[2] Choudhary A, Wright L, Ponce O, Chen J, Prashar A, Sanchez-Moran E, et al. Varietal variation and chromosome behavior during meiosis in *Solanum tuberosum*. Heredity. 2020;**125**:212-226. DOI: 10.1038/s41437-020-0328-6

[3] Braynen J, Yang Y, Yuan J, Xie Z, Cao G, Wei X, et al. Comparative transcriptome analysis revealed differential gene expression in multiple signaling pathways at flowering in polyploidy *Brassica rapa*. Cell & Bioscience. 2021;**11**:17. DOI: 10.1186/s13578-021-00528-1

[4] Abberton M, Batley J, Bentley A, Bryant J, Cai H, Cockram J, et al. Global agricultural intensification during climate change: A role for genomics. Plant Biotechnology Journal. 2016;**14**: 1095-1098. DOI: 10.1111/pbi.12467

[5] Touchell DH, Palmer IE, Ranney TG. *In vitro* ploidy manipulation for crop improvement. Frontiers in Plant Science. 2020;**11**:722. DOI: 10.3389/fpls.2020.00722

[6] Storme ND, Mason A. Plant speciation through chromosome instability and ploidy change: Cellular mechanisms, molecular factors and evolutionary relevance. Current Plant Biology. 2014;**1**:10-33

[7] Machida-Hirano R. Diversity of potato genetic resources. Breeding Science. 2015;**65**:26-40. DOI: 10.1270/jsbbs.65.26

[8] Hawkes JG. The potato: Evolution, biodiversity and genetic resources. American Potato Journal. 1990;**67**: 733-735. DOI: 10.1007/BF03044023

[9] Watanabe KN. Potato genetics, genomics, and applications. Breeding Science. 2015;**65**:53-68. DOI: 10.1270/jsbbs.65.53

[10] Muthoni J, Kabira J, Shimelis H, Melis R. Tetrasomic inheritance in cultivated potato and implications in conventional breeding. Australian Journal of Crop Science. 2015;**9**:185-190

[11] Jansky SH, Spooner DM. The evolution of potato breeding. Plant Breeding Reviews. 2018;**41**:169-214. DOI: 10.1002/9781119414735

[12] Olvera-Vazquez S, Cadena-Iñiguez J, Gilani S, Watanabe K. The cytological studies on neglected and underutilized cucurbit species with special reference to Chayote, an under-exploited species. American Journal of Plant Sciences. 2019;**10**(8):1261-1279. DOI: 10.4236/ajps.2019.108091

[13] Lira-Saade R. Chayote. Sechiumedule (Jacq.) Sw. Promoting the Conservation and Use of Underutilized and Neglected Crops. Rome: Institute of Plant Genetics and Crop Plant Research; 1996

[14] De Donato M, Cequea H. A cytogenetic study of six cultivars of the Chayote, *Sechium edule* Sw. (Cucurbitaceae). Journal of Heredity. 1994;**85**:238-241. DOI: 10.1093/oxfordjournals.jhered.a111444

[15] Mercado P, Lira R. Contribucion al conocimiento de los numerous cromosomicos de los generos Sechium P. BR. Y Sicana Naudin (*Cucurbitaceae*). Acta Botanica Mexicana. 1994;**27**:7-13. DOI: 10.21829/abm27.1994.706

[16] Bisognin DA. Origin and evolution of cultivated cucurbits. Ciencia Rural. 2002;**32**:715-723. DOI: 10.1590/S0103-84782002000400028

[17] Varghese RM. Cytology of *Sechium edule* Sw. Current Science. 1973;**42**:30

[18] eFloras. 11. *Curcuma* Linnaeus. In: Flora of China. Vol. Vol. 24. St. Louis, MO/Cambridge, MA: Missouri Botanical Garden/Harvard University Herbaria; 2020. p. 359. Available from: http://www.efloras.org

[19] Wu DL, Larsen K. Zingiberaceae. In: Wu ZY, Raven P, Hong DY, editors. Flora of China. Vol. 24. Beijing, China/ St. Louis, MO: Science Press/Missouri Botanical Garden Press; 2000. pp. 322-377

[20] Leong-Skornickova J, Newman M. Gingers of Cambodia, Laos and Vietnam. Singapore: Singapore Botanic Gardens; 2015

[21] Larsen K. A preliminary checklist of the *Zingiberaceae* of Thailand. Thai Forest Bulletin (Botany). 1996;**24**:35-49

[22] Leong-Skornickova J, Sida O, Jarolimova V, Sabu M, Fer T, Travnicek P, et al. Chromosome numbers and genome size variation in Indian species of *Curcuma* (Zingiberaceae). Annals of Botany. 2007;**100**:505-526

[23] Maknoi C. Taxonomy and phylogeny of the genus *Curcuma* L. (Zingiberaceae) with particular reference to its occurrence in Thailand [PhD thesis]. Thailand: Prince of Songkla University; 2006

[24] eFloras. 20. Zingiberaceae Lindley. In: Flora of China. Vol. Vol. 24. St. Louis, MO/Cambridge, MA: Missouri Botanical Garden/Harvard University Herbaria; 2020. p. 322. Available from: http://www.efloras.org

[25] Hojsgaard D, Honfi AI, Rua G, Daviña J. Chromosome numbers and ploidy levels of *Paspalum* species from subtropical South America (Poaceae). Genetic Resources and Crop Evolution. 2009;**56**:533-545. DOI: 10.1007/s10722-008-9384-0

[26] Hodálová I, Mered'ajun P, Vinikarová A, Grulich V, Rotreklová O. A new cytotype of *Jacobaea vulgaris* (Asteraceae): Frequency, morphology and origin. Nordic Journal of Botany. 2010;**28**:413-427. DOI: 10.1111/j.1756-1051.2010.00603.x

[27] Gu AX, Zhao JJ, Li LM, Wang YH, Zhao YJ, Hua F, et al. Analyses of phenotype and ARGOS and ASY1 expression in a ploidy Chinese cabbage series derived from one haploid. Breeding Science. 2016;**66**(2):161-168. DOI: 10.1270/jsbbs.66.161

[28] Wang B, Sang Y, Song J, Gao XQ, Zhang X. Expression of a rice *OsARGOS* gene in *Arabidopsis* promotes cell division and expansion and increases organ size. Journal of Genetics and Genomics. 2009;**36**(1):31-40. DOI: 10.1016/s1673-8527(09)60004-7

[29] Allario T, Brumos J, Colmenero-Flores JM, Tadeo F, Froelicher Y, Talon M, et al. Large changes in anatomy and physiology between diploid Rangpur lime (*Citrus limonia*) and its autotetraploid are not associated with large changes in leaf gene expression. Journal of Experimental Botany. 2011;**62**(8):2507-2519. DOI: 10.1093/jxb/erq467

[30] Qiao G, Liu M, Song K, Li H, Yang H, Yin Y, et al. Phenotypic and comparative transcriptome analysis of different ploidy plants in *Dendrocalamus latiflorus* Munro. Frontiers in Plant Science. 2017;**8**:1371. DOI: 10.3389/fpls.2017.01371

[31] Bird D, Beisson F, Brigham A, Shin J, Greer S, Jetter R, et al. Characterization of *Arabidopsis* ABCG11/WBC11, an ATP binding cassette (ABC) transporter that is required for cuticular lipid secretion. Plant Journal. 2007;**52**(3):485-498. DOI: 10.1111/j.1365-313X.2007.03252.x

[32] Narukawa H, Yokoyama R, Komaki S, Sugimoto K, Nishitani K. Stimulation of cell elongation by tetraploidy in hypocotyls of dark grown

Arabidopsis seedlings. PLoS One. 2015;**10**(8):e0134547. DOI: 10.1371/journal.pone.0134547

[33] Narukawa H, Yokoyama R, Nishitani K. Possible pathways linking ploidy level to cell elongation and cuticular function in hypocotyls of dark-grown *Arabidopsis* seedlings. Plant Signaling & Behavior. 2016;**11**(2): e1118597. DOI: 10.1080/15592324.2015.1118597

[34] Zhou Y, Kang L, Liao S, Pan Q, Ge X, Li Z. Transcriptomic analysis reveals differential gene expressions for cell growth and functional secondary metabolites in induced autotetraploid of Chinese woad (*Isatis indigotica* fort.). PLoS One. 2015;**10**(3):e0116392. DOI: 10.1371/journal.pone.0116392

[35] Wang Z, Fan G, Dong Y, Zhai X, Deng M, Zhao Z, et al. Implications of polyploidy events on the phenotype, microstructure, and proteome of *Paulownia australis*. PLoS One. 2017;**12**(3):e0172633. DOI: 10.1371/journal.pone.0172633

[36] Lavania UC, Srivastava S, Lavania S, Basu S, Misra NK, Mukai Y. Autopolyploidy differentially influences body size in plants, but facilitates enhanced accumulation of secondary metabolites, causing increased cytosine methylation. The Plant Journal. 2012;**71**(4):539-549. DOI: 10.1111/j.1365-313X.2012.05006.x

[37] Ding M, Chen ZJ. Epigenetic perspectives on the evolution and domestication of polyploid plant and crops. Current Opinion in Plant Biology. 2018;**42**:37-48. DOI: 10.1016/j.pbi.2018.02.003

[38] Doyle JJ, Coate JE. Polyploidy, the nucleotype, and novelty: The impact of genome doubling on the biology of the cell. International Journal of Plant Sciences. 2019;**180**(1):1-52. DOI: 10.1086/700636

[39] Alam H, Razaq M, Salahuddin. Induced polyploidy as a tool for increasing tea (*Camellia sinensis* L.) production. Journal of Northeast Agricultural University (English Edition). 2015;**22**(3):43-47. DOI: 10.1016/S1006-8104(16)30005-8

[40] Eliášová A, Műnzbergová Z. Higher seed size and germination rate may favor autotetraploids of *Vicia cracca* L. (Fabaceae). Biological Journal of the Linnean Society. 2014;**113**:57-73

[41] Mu H, Liu Z, Lin L, Li H, Jiang J, Liu G. Transcriptomic analysis of phenotypic changes in birch (*Betula platyphylla*) autotetraploids. International Journal of Molecular Sciences. 2012;**13**(10):13012-13029. DOI: 10.3390/ijms131013012

[42] Ma Y, Xue H, Zhang L, Zhang F, Ou C, Wang F, et al. Involvement of auxin and brassinosteroid in dwarfism of autotetraploid apple (*Malus* × *domestica*). Scientific Reports. 2016;**6**:26719. DOI: 10.1038/srep26719

[43] Gantait S, Mukherjee E. Induced autopolyploidy—A promising approach for enhanced biosynthesis of plant secondary metabolites: An insight. Genetic Engineering and Biotechnology. 2021;**19**:4. DOI: 10.1186/s43141-020-00109-8

[44] Mishra B, Pathak S, Sharma A, Trivedi P, Shukla S. Modulated gene expression in newly synthesized autotetraploid of *Papaver somniferum* L. South African Journal of Botany. 2010;**76**(3):447-452. DOI: 10.1016/j.sajb.2010.02.090

[45] Vergara F, Kikuchi J, Breuer C. Artificial autopolyploidization modifies the tricarboxylic acid cycle and GABA shunt in *Arabidopsis thaliana* Col-0. Scientific Reports. 2016;**6**:26515. DOI: 10.1038/srep26515

[46] Dou J, Yuan P, Zhao S, He N, Zhu H, Gao L, et al. Effect of ploidy level on

expression of lycopene biosynthesis genes and accumulation of phytohormones during watermelon (*Citrullus lanatus*) fruit development and ripening. Journal of Integrative Agriculture. 2017;**16**(9):19561967. DOI: 10.1016/S2095-3119(16)61618-0

[47] Javadian N, Karimzadeh G, Sharifi M, Moieni A, Behmanesh M. *In vitro* polyploidy induction: Changes in morphology, podophyllotoxin biosynthesis, and expression of the related genes in *Linum album* (*Linaceae*). Planta. 2017;**245**(6):1165-1178. DOI: 10.1007/s00425-017-2671-2

[48] Amah D, van Biljon A, Maziya-Dixon B, Labuschagne M, Swennen R. Effects of in vitro polyploidization on agronomic characteristics and fruit carotenoid content: Implications for banana genetic improvement. Frontiers in Plant Science. 2019;**10**:1450. DOI: 10.3389/fpls.2019.01450

[49] Chung HH, Shi SK, Huang B, Chen JT. Enhanced agronomic traits and medicinal constituents of autotetraploids in *Anoectochilus formosanus* Hayata, a top-grade medicinal orchid. Molecules. 2017;**22**(11). DOI: 10.3390/molecules22111907

[50] Preet R, Gupta RC. Fatty acid profiling in diploid (n=12) and tetraploid cytotypes (n=24) of *Physalis angulata* Linn. from Rajasthan by gas chromatography. International Journal of Pharmaceutical Sciences and Research. 2017;**8**(8):3458-3462

[51] Catalano C, Abbate L, Motisi A, Crucitti D, Cangelosi V, Pisciotta A, et al. Autotetraploid emergence via somatic embryogenesis in *Vitis vinifera* induces marked morphological changes in shoots, mature leaves, and stomata. Cell. 2021;**10**:1336. DOI: 10.3390/cells10061336

[52] Sattler MC, Carvalho CR, Clarindo WR. The polyploidy and its key role in plant breeding. Planta. 2015. DOI: 10.1007/s00425-015-2450-x

[53] Ruiz M, Oustric J, Santini J, Morillon R. Synthetic polyploidy in grafted crops. Frontiers in Plant Science. 2020;**11**:540894. DOI: 10.3389/fpls.2020.540894

[54] Meng H, Jiang S, Hua S, Lin X, Li Y, Guo W, et al. Comparison between a tetraploid turnip and its diploid progenitor (*Brassica rapa* L.): The adaptation to salinity stress. Agricultural Sciences in China. 2013;**10**(3):363-375. DOI: 10.1016/S1671-2927(11)60015-1

[55] Tu Y, Jiang A, Gan L, Hossain M, Zhang J, Peng B, et al. Genome duplication improves rice root resistance to salt stress. Rice. 2014;**7**(1):15-15. DOI: 10.1186/s12284-014-0015-4

[56] Xue H, Zhang F, Zhang Z, Fu J, Wang F, Zhang B, et al. Differences in salt tolerance between diploid and autotetraploid apple seedlings exposed to salt stress. Scientia Horticulturae. 2015;**190**:24-30. DOI: 10.1016/j.scienta.2015.04.009

[57] Yan K, Wu C, Zhang L, Chen X. Contrasting photosynthesis and photoinhibition in tetraploid and its autodiploid honeysuckle (*Lonicera japonica* Thunb.) under salt stress. Frontiers in Plant Science. 2015;**6**:227. DOI: 10.3389/fpls.2015.00227

[58] Fan G, Li X, Deng M, Zhao Z, Yang L. Comparative analysis and identification of miRNAs and their target genes responsive to salt stress in diploid and tetraploid *Paulownia fortunei* seedlings. PLoS One. 2016;**11**(2):e0149617. DOI: 10.1371/journal.pone.0149617

[59] Fan G, Wang L, Deng M, Zhao Z, Dong Y, Zhang X, et al. Changes in transcript related to osmosis and intracellular ion homeostasis in

Paulownia tomentosa under salt stress. Frontiers in Plant Science. 2016;7:384. DOI: 10.3389/fpls.2016.00384

[60] Yu L, Liu X, Boge W, Liu X. Genome-wide association study identifies loci for salt tolerance during germination in autotetraploid alfalfa (*Medicago sativa* L.) using genotyping by-sequencing. Frontiers in Plant Science. 2016;7:956. DOI: 10.3389/fpls.2016.00956

[61] Deng M, Dong Y, Zhao Z, Li Y, Fan G. Dissecting the proteome dynamics of the salt stress induced changes in the leaf of diploid and autotetraploid *Paulownia fortunei*. PLoS One. 2017;**12**(7):e0181937. DOI: 10.1371/journal.pone.0181937

[62] Liu B, Sun G. microRNAs contribute to enhanced salt adaptation of the autopolyploid *Hordeum bulbosum* compared with its diploid ancestor. Plant Journal. 2017;**91**(1):57-69. DOI: 10.1111/tpj.13546

[63] Zhao Z, Li Y, Liu H, Zhai X, Deng M, Dong Y, et al. Genome-wide expression analysis of salt-stressed diploid and autotetraploid *Paulownia tomentosa*. PLoS One. 2017;**12**(10): e0185455. DOI: 10.1371/journal.pone.0185455

[64] del Pozo JC, Ramirez-Parra E. Deciphering the molecular bases for drought tolerance in *Arabidopsis* autotetraploids. Plant, Cell and Environment. 2014;**37**(12):2722-2737. DOI: 10.1111/pce.12344

[65] Niu S, Wang Y, Zhao Z, Deng M, Cao L, Yang L, et al. Transcriptome and degradome of microRNAs and their targets in response to drought stress in the plants of a diploid and its autotetraploid *Paulownia australis*. PLoS One. 2016;**11**(7):e0158750. DOI: 10.1371/journal.pone.0158750

[66] Cao X, Fan G, Cao L, Deng M, Zhao Z, Niu S, et al. Drought stress-induced changes of microRNAs in diploid and autotetraploid *Paulownia tomentosa*. Genes & Genomics. 2017;**39**(1):77-86. DOI: 10.1007/s13258-016-0473-8

[67] Zhao Z, Niu S, Fan G, Deng M, Wang Y. Genome-wide analysis of gene and microRNA expression in diploid and autotetraploid *Paulownia fortunei* (Seem) Hemsl. under drought stress by transcriptome, microRNA, and degradome sequencing. Forests. 2018;**9**(2):88. DOI: 10.3390/f9020088

[68] Rao S, Tian Y, Xia X, Li Y, Chen J. Chromosome doubling mediates superior drought tolerance in *Lycium ruthenicum* via abscisic acid signaling. Horticulture Research. 2020;7:40. DOI: 10.1038/s41438-020-0260-1

[69] Li M, Zhang C, Hou L, Yang W, Liu S, Pang X, et al. Multiple responses contribute to the enhanced drought tolerance of the autotetraploid *Ziziphus jujuba* Mill. var. *spinosa*. Cell & Bioscience. 2021;**11**:119. DOI: 10.1186/s13578-021-00633-1

[70] Zhang XY, Hu CG, Yao JL. Tetraploidization of diploid *Dioscorea* results in activation of the antioxidant defense system and increased heat tolerance. Journal of Plant Physiology. 2010;**167**(2):88-94. DOI: 10.1016/j.jplph.2009.07.006

[71] DeBolt S. Copy number variation shapes genome diversity in *Arabidopsis* over immediate family generational scales. Genome Biology and Evolution. 2010;**2**:441-453. DOI: 10.1093/gbe/evq033

[72] Deng B, Du W, Changlai L, Sun W, Tian S, Dong H. Antioxidant response to drought, cold and nutrient stress in two ploidy levels of tobacco plants: Low resource requirement confers polytolerance in polyploids. Plant Growth Regulation. 2012;**66**(1):37-47. DOI: 10.1007/s10725-011-9626-6

[73] Syngelaki E, Daubert M, Klatt S, Hörandl E. Phenotypic responses,

reproduction mode and epigenetic patterns under temperature treatments in the alpine plant species *Ranunculus kuepferi* (*Ranunculaceae*). Biology. 2020;**9**:315. DOI: 10.3390/biology 9100315

[74] Ruiz M, Quiñones A, Martínez Alcántara B, Aleza P, Morillon R, Navarro L, et al. Tetraploidy enhances boron-excess tolerance in Carrizo Citrange (*Citrus sinensis* L. Osb. × *Poncirus trifoliata* L. Raf.). Frontiers in Plant Science. 2016;7:701. DOI: 10.3389/ fpls.2016.00701

[75] Li M, Xu G, Xia X, Wang M, Yin X, Zhang B, et al. Deciphering the physiological and molecular mechanisms for copper tolerance in autotetraploid *Arabidopsis*. Plant Cell Reports. 2017;**36**(10):1585-1597. DOI: 10.1007/s00299-017-2176-2

[76] Mu H, Lin L, Zhang Q, Tang X, Zhang X, Cheng G. Growth, proline content and proline-associated gene expression of autotetraploid *Betula platyphylla* responding to $NaHCO_3$ stress. Dendrobiology. 2016;**75**:123-129. DOI: 10.12657/denbio.075.012

[77] Hias N, Svara A, Wannes Keulemans J. Effect of polyploidisation on the response of apple (*Malus* × *domestica* Borkh.) to *Venturia inaequalis* infection. European Journal of Plant Pathology. 2018;**151**(2):515-526. DOI: 10.1007/s10658-017-1395-2

[78] Jansky S, Haynes K, Douches D. Comparison of two strategies to introgress genes for resistance to common scab from diploid *Solanum chacoense* into tetraploid cultivated potato. American Journal of Potato Research. 2019;**96**:255-261. DOI: 10.1007/s12230-018-09711-6

[79] Ramsey J, Ramsey TS. Ecological studies of polyploidy in the 100 years following its discovery. Philosophical Transactions of the Royal Society B. 2014;**369**:20130352. DOI: 10.1098/ rstb.2013.0352

[80] Makarevitch I, Harris C. Aneuploidy causes tissue-specific qualitative changes in global gene expression patterns in maize. Plant Physiology. 2010;**152**:927-938. DOI: 10.1104/pp.109.150466

[81] Spoelhof JP, Soltis PS, Soltis DE. Pure polyploidy: Closing the gaps in autopolyploid research. Journal of Systematics and Evolution. 2017;**55**(4): 340-352. DOI: 10.1111/jse.12253

[82] Bohutínská M, Alston M, Monnahan P, Mandáková T, Bray S, Paajanen P, et al. Novelty and convergence in adaptation to whole genome duplication. Molecular Biology and Evolution. 2021:msab096. DOI: 10.1093/molbev/msab096

[83] Baduel P, Quadrana L, Hunter B, Bomblies K, Colot V. Relaxed purifying selection in autopolyploids drives transposable element overaccumulation which provides variants for local adaptation. Nature Communications. 2019;**10**:5818. DOI: 10.1038/ s41467-019-13730-0

[84] Hurka H, Bleeker W, Neuffer B. Evolutionary processes associated with biological invasions in the Brassicaceae. Biological Invasions. 2003;**5**:281-292

[85] Kubátová B, Trávníček P, Bastlová D, Čurn V, Jarolímová V, Suda J. DNA ploidy-level variation in native and invasive populations of *Lythrum salicaria* at a large geographical scale. Journal of Biogeography. 2008;**35**: 167-176

[86] del Rio AH, Bamberg JB. Detection of adaptive genetic diversity in wild potato populations and its implications in conservation of potato germplasm. American Journal of Plant Sciences. 2020;**11**:1562-1578. DOI: 10.4236/ ajps.2020.1110113

[87] Fox DT, Soltis DE, Soltis PS, Ashman TL, de Peer YV. Polyploidy: A biological force from cells to ecosystems. Trends in Cell Biology. 2020. DOI: 10.1016/j.tcb.2020.06.006

[88] Campos H, Ortiz O. The Potato Crop: Its Agricultural, Nutritional and Social Contribution to Humankind2020. DOI: 10.1007/978-3-030-28683-5

[89] Stenberg P, Saura A. Meiosis and its deviations in polyploid animals. Cytogenetic and Genome Research. 2013;**140**:185-203. DOI: 10.1159/000351731

[90] Comai L. The advantages and disadvantages of being polyploid. Nature. 2005;**6**:836-846. DOI: 10.1038/nrg1711

Section 3

Study of Sociodemographic Factors and Causes of Down Syndrome

Chapter 4

Study on the Effect of Socio-Demographic Factors on Different Congenital Disorders

Poulami Majumder and Subrata Kumar Dey

Abstract

Congenital disorders define the disease that occurs since the birth of a baby. Down syndrome, Turner syndrome, cleft lip, and congenital heart disease are the most common congenital disorders worldwide. A retrospective study was carried out, examining the effect of sociodemographic factors on congenital anomalies in the state of West Bengal, India, over a period of 6 years. A total of 595 cases with congenital disorders including Down syndrome, Turner syndrome, and other abnormalities (cleft lip/palate, syndactyly, ambiguous genitalia) were statistically analyzed along with the sociodemographic characteristics through Statistical Analysis System (SAS) 9.3.2. Down syndrome is seemed to be associated with age, ethnicity, parental addiction, especially smoking, while Turner syndrome is associated with ethnicity and gender. Other congenital disorders such as ambiguous genitalia are found to be associated with maternal addiction.

Keywords: congenital disorders, down syndrome, turner syndrome, cleft lip/palate, syndactyly, ambiguous genitalia, sociodemographic factors

1. Introduction

Congenital disorder, which is a health hazard since birth, may be caused mostly by genetic anomalies [1]. Some congenital disorders are hereditary that are transmitted through parents to the children [2]. Several types of congenital disorders are present of which the most common congenital disorders are Down syndrome, Turner syndrome, congenital heart diseases, etc., are considered the most common and severe disorders since birth [3–5]. This type of disorder cannot be cured but managed, though some of them can be prevented or cured such as cleft lip/palate through surgical intervention [6]. The exact cause of congenital abnormalities is not fully understood. Sometimes it depends on genetic or infectious factors, and sometimes it may be caused by nutritional or environmental factors [7–9].

In this book chapter, we have discussed the possible effect of sociodemographic factors, including environmental and behavioral facets on congenital disorders [10]. The main focused congenital disorders are Down syndrome (2n = 47, XX/XY, +21) and Turner syndrome (2n = 45, X). Down syndrome is a genetic condition with an extra chromosome (chromosome no. 21) that presents since birth and this condition results in developmental delay along with associated diseases such as heart disease, intestinal obstruction [11–13]. This "package" of the 21st chromosome (trisomy or three copies of chromosome 21) is caused due to nondisjunction of chromosome 21 in meiotic cell division during the development of the sperm cell or the egg cell [14]. Studies suggest that the advanced maternal age, the addiction of the mother as well as the father may be the prime cause for this kind of condition to their child [15, 16]. However, sociodemographic factors are also thought to be associated with these diseases [17]. Another common congenital disorder is Turner syndrome, which is also discussed in this chapter. Turner syndrome only affects females and one of the X chromosomes (sex chromosome) is fully or partially missing [18]. This condition results in a variety of medical and developmental problems such as short stature, webbed neck, delayed development of ovaries, heart defects, loss of puberty and menstruation, infertility [19]. Most of the cases of Turner syndrome cannot be cured, though hormone therapy can be useful for treatment in some cases [20]. Turner syndrome occurs due to the nondisjunction of the X chromosome in meiotic cell division during the formation of an egg or sperm cell in a parent (prior to conception) [21]. The other discussed congenital anomalies include cleft lip/palate, syndactyly, and ambiguous genitalia. Cleft lip/palate is a common birth condition. It occurs alone or as part of a genetic condition or syndrome [22, 23]. Symptoms arise from the opening in the mouth and include the difficulty in speaking and feeding [24]. Surgeries are the useful treatment for this condition [25]. Sometimes speech therapy helps to improve the speaking ability [26]. Syndactyly is the fusion of the bone or skin in the hand or foot digits [27]. This condition is due to developmental anomalies. Ambiguous genitalia is a rare condition in which an infant's external genitals do not appear to be clearly manifested as a either male or female [28]. In a baby with ambiguous external genitalia, the genitals may be incompletely developed or the baby may have characteristics of both sexes [29]. Karyotype helps in determining the proper sex of the patients and subsequent surgical intervention is required to cure the affected individuals.

The sociodemographic features involve a combination of social and demographic facets. Social facets include behavioral factors such as addiction where the demographic part includes age, gender, race, etc. [30]. This work is a descriptive analysis of all different sociodemographic factors, including other diseases, associated with studied congenital disorders.

2. Materials and methods

Data were collected from a retrospective study, examining the sociodemographic factors along with a few behavioral characteristics from the state of West Bengal, India, along with the diagnostic information about common congenital disorders for the 595 samples over a period of 6 years (2011–2017). Patients were diagnosed at the Centre for Genetic Studies, Maulana Abul Kalam Azad University of Technology. All data were recorded after taking the informed consent from the participants. Collected data were entered using a database mamgement software MySQL. Entered data were exported to SAS (Statistical Analysis Software version 9.3.2) and analyzed for understanding the patterns and predictors of the identified genetic disorders. Descriptive analyses were conducted to determine the frequency and proportion (along with corresponding 95% confidence intervals and p values to denote whether the categories for each factor had a statistically significant different distribution of the proportions) of the sociodemographic factors (gender, religion), behavioral factors (consanguinity, contraception use, addiction), clinical history (history of spontaneous abortion, diabetes, hormonal deficiency), family history (history of congenital abnormalities among relatives and disease distribution if any such as Down, Turner, and other congenital abnormalities) among the sampled population. The sum of the total frequencies in all the categories in each variable will not be equal to 595 as there were multiple missing values for different variables and while analyzing the distribution and associations, they were dropped. Binary and multinomial, and logistic regressions were next conducted to determine the association (odds ratios, corresponding 95% confidence intervals, and p values) between the study variables and diagnosed diseases. Multiple logistic regressions to determine the association between the variables adjusted for all others could not be done for inadequate sample size. The results of the analyses are presented in **Tables 1–9**. Each table is followed immediately by the interpretation of the observed results presented in each of these tables, respectively.

Variables	Categories	N	95% CI	P value
Gender	Male	279	46.89 (42.87–50.91)	<.0001
	Female	313	52.61 (48.58–56.63)	
Religion	Muslim	152	28.52 (24.67–32.36)	<.0001
	Hindu	381	71.48 (67.64–75.33)	
History of consanguinity	Yes	28	4.71 (3.00–6.41)	<.0001
	No	567	95.29 (93.59–97.00)	
Contraceptives used	Yes	104	17.48 (14.42–20.54)	<.0001
	No	491	82.52 (79.46–85.58)	
Addiction of father	None	341	57.31 (53.33–61.30)	<.0001
	Smoking	178	29.92 (26.23–33.61)	
	Smoking/drug	65	10.92 (8.41–13.44)	
	Smoking/drug/alcohol	11	1.85 (0.76–2.93)	
History of spontaneous abortion	Yes	206	86.19 (81.79–90.60)	<.0001
	No	33	13.81 (9.40–18.21)	
Presence of diabetes	Yes	43	7.23 (5.14–9.31)	<.0001
	No	552	92.77 (90.69–94.86)	
Presence of hormonal deficiencies (FSH/TSH/etc.)	Yes	62	10.42 (7.96–12.88)	<.0001
	No	533	89.58 (87.12–92.04)	
History of congenital disease among first degree relatives	Yes	71	11.93 (9.32–14.55)	<.0001
	No	524	88.07 (85.46–90.68)	
Any genetic abnormality detected	No	308	51.76 (47.74–55.79)	0.3893
	Yes	287	48.24 (44.21–52.26)	
Down syndrome	Neither Down nor Mosaic	331	55.63 (51.63–59.63)	<.0001
	Down syndrome	254	42.69 (38.70–46.67)	
	Mosaic Down syndrome	10	1.68 (0.64–2.72)	
Turner syndrome	Yes	11	1.85 (0.76–2.93)	<.0001
	No	584	98.15 (97.07–99.24)	
Child with congenital abnormalities	Yes	11	1.85 (0.76–2.93)	<.0001
	No	584	98.15 (97.07–99.24)	

Table 1.
Descriptive analyses of the samples analyzed (n = 595).

Variables	Categories	Yes			No		
		N	95% CI	P value	N	95% CI	P value
Gender	Male	5	45.45 (10.37–80.54)	0.7630	274	46.92 (42.86–50.98)	<.0001
	Female	6	54.55 (19.46–89.63)		307	52.57 (48.51–56.63)	
Religion	Muslim	2	25.00 (0.00–63.70)	0.1573	150	28.57 (24.69–32.45)	<.0001
	Hindu	6	75.00 (36.30–100.00)		375	71.43 (67.55–75.31)	
History of consanguinity	Yes	1	9.09 (0.00–29.35)	0.0067	27	4.62 (2.92–6.33)	<.0001
	No	10	90.91 (70.65–100.00)		557	95.38 (93.67–97.08)	
Contraceptives used	Yes	3	27.27 (0.00–58.65)	0.1317	101	17.29 (14.22–20.37)	<.0001
	No	8	72.73 (41.35–100.00)		483	82.71 (79.63–85.78)	
Addiction of father	None	8	72.73 (41.35–100.00)	0.0201	333	57.02 (52.99–61.05)	<.0001
	Smoking	2	18.18 (0.00–45.36)		176	30.14 (26.40–33.87)	
	Smoking/ Drug	1	9.09 (0.00–29.35)		64	10.96 (8.42–13.50)	
	Smoking,/ Drug/ Alcohol	—	—	—	11	1.88 (0.78–2.99)	
History of spontaneous abortion	Yes	4	80.00 (24.47–100.00)	0.1797	202	86.32 (81.89–90.76)	<.0001
	No	1	20.00 (0.00–75.53)		32	13.68 (9.24–18.11)	
Presence of diabetes	Yes	1	9.09 (0.00–29.35)	0.0067	42	7.19 (5.09–9.29)	<.0001
	No	10	90.91 (70.65–100.00)		542	92.81 (90.71–94.91)	
Presence of hormonal deficiencies (FSH/TSH/ etc.)	Yes	2	18.18 (0.00–45.36)	0.0348	60	10.27 (7.80–12.74)	<.0001
	No	9	81.82 (54.64–100.00)		524	89.73 (87.26–92.20)	
History of congenital disease among first-degree relative	Yes	1	9.09 (0.00–29.35)	0.0067	70	11.99 (9.34–14.63)	<.0001
	No	10	90.91 (70.65–100.00)		514	88.01 (85.37–90.66)	
Any genetic abnormality detected	Yes	7	63.64 (29.74–97.53)	0.3657	301	51.54 (47.48–55.61)	0.4564
	No	4	36.36 (2.47–70.26)		283	48.46 (44.39–52.52)	
Down syndrome	Neither down nor Mosaic	7	63.64 (29.74–97.53)	0.3657	324	55.48 (51.44–59.52)	<.0001
	Down syndrome	4	36.36 (2.47–70.26)		250	42.81 (38.78–46.83)	
	Mosaic Down syndrome	—	—	—	10	1.71 (0.66–2.77)	
Turner syndrome	Yes	—	—	—	11	1.88 (0.78–2.99)	<.0001
	No	11	100.00 (100.00–100.00)	—	573	98.12 (97.01–99.22)	

Table 2.
Descriptive analyses regarding congenital anomalies.

3. Results

The tablewise description is as follows:

In **Table 1**: of the total 595 samples analyzed, 279 (46.89%) were males, 313 (52.61%) were females, and for three subjects sex could not be determined. The majority belonged to the Hindu religion (381, 71.48%) followed by Muslim (152, 28.52%). A history of consanguinity was observed among 28 (4.71%) subjects. Among females who got pregnant, 206 (86.19%) had a history of spontaneous abortion and 104 (17.48%) reported use of contraceptives, 178 (29.92%) fathers were addicted to smoking, 65 (10.92%) to both smoking and drugs, and 11 (1.85%) to either smoking or drugs or alcohol. Among total subjects, 43 (7.23%) were diagnosed with diabetes, 62 (10.42%) had some hormonal deficiencies, and 71 (11.93%) had a history of congenital disease among first-degree relatives. More than half of the tested samples [308 (51.76%)] were from normal subjects, 254 (42.69%)

Variables	Categories	Any genetic abnormality detected					
		No			Yes		
		N	95% CI	P value	N	95% CI	P value
Gender	Male	116	37.66 (32.22–43.10)	<.0001	163	56.79 (51.03–62.56)	<.0001
	Female	190	61.69 (56.23–67.15)		123	42.86 (37.10–48.62)	
Religion	Muslim	73	28.40 (22.85–33.96)	<.0001	79	28.62 (23.26–33.99)	<.0001
	Hindu	184	71.60 (66.04–77.15)		197	71.38 (66.01–76.74)	
History of consanguinity	Yes	15	4.87 (2.45–7.29)	<.0001	13	4.53 (2.11–6.95)	<.0001
	No	293	95.13 (92.71–97.55)		274	95.47 (93.05–97.89)	
Contraceptives Used	Yes	48	15.58 (11.51–19.66)	<.0001	56	19.51 (14.90–24.12)	<.0001
	No	260	84.42 (80.34–88.49)		231	80.49 (75.88–85.10)	
Addiction of father	None	181	58.77 (53.24–64.29)	<.0001	160	55.75 (49.97–61.53)	<.0001
	Smoking	93	30.19 (25.04–35.35)		85	29.62 (24.30–34.93)	
	Smoking/ drug	27	8.77 (5.59–11.94)		38	13.24 (9.30–17.19)	
	Smoking/ drug/ alcohol	7	2.27 (0.60–3.95)		4	1.39 (0.03–2.76)	
History of spontaneous abortion	Yes	104	80.62 (73.71–87.53)	<.0001	102	92.73 (87.80–97.66)	<.0001
	No	25	19.38 (12.47–26.29)		8	7.27 (2.34–12.20)	
Presence of diabetes	Yes	21	6.82 (3.99–9.65)	<.0001	22	7.67 (4.57–10.76)	<.0001
	No	287	93.18 (90.35–96.01)		265	92.33 (89.24–95.43)	
Presence of hormonal deficiencies (FSH/TSH/etc.)	Yes	29	9.42 (6.14–12.70)	<.0001	33	11.50 (7.79–15.21)	<.0001
	No	279	90.58 (87.30–93.86)		254	88.50 (84.79–92.21)	
History of congenital disease among first-degree relative	Yes	39	12.66 (8.93–16.40)	<.0001	32	11.15 (7.49–14.81)	<.0001
	No	269	87.34 (83.60–91.07)		255	88.85 (85.19–92.51)	

Table 3.
Descriptive analyses regarding congenital abnormalities.

Variables	Categories	Diagnosed with								
		Neither Down nor Mosaic (n = 331)			Down syndrome (n = 254)			Mosaic Down syndrome (n = 10)		
		N	95% CI	p value	N	95% CI	P value	N	95% CI	P value
Gender	Male	119	35.95 (30.76–41.15)	<.0001	155	61.02 (54.99–67.06)	0.0004	5	50.00 (12.30–87.70)	1.0000
	Female	209	63.14 (57.92–68.37)		99	38.98 (32.94–45.01)		5	50.00 (12.30–87.70)	
Religion	Muslim	82	29.50 (24.10–34.89)	<.0001	68	27.76 (22.11–33.40)	<.0001	2	20.00 (0.00–50.16)	0.0578
	Hindu	196	70.50 (65.11–75.90)		177	72.24 (66.60–77.89)		8	80.00 (49.84–100.00)	
History of consanguinity	Yes	15	4.53 (2.28–6.78)	<.0001	11	4.33 (1.81–6.85)	<.0001	2	20.00 (0.00–50.16)	0.0578
	No	316	95.47 (93.22–97.72)		243	95.67 (93.15–98.19)		8	80.00 (49.84–100.00)	
Contraceptives used	Yes	52	15.71 (11.77–19.65)	<.0001	49	19.29 (14.41–24.18)	<.0001	3	30.00 (0.00–64.56)	0.2059
	No	279	84.29 (80.35–88.23)		205	80.71 (75.82–85.59)		7	70.00 (35.45–100.00)	
Addiction of father	None	191	57.70 (52.35–63.05)	<.0001	147	57.87 (51.76–63.99)	<.0001	3	30.00 (0.00–64.56)	0.9048
	Smoking	101	30.51 (25.53–35.50)		73	28.74 (23.14–34.34)		4	40.00 (3.06–76.94)	
	Smoking/drug	31	9.37 (6.21–12.52)		31	12.20 (8.15–16.26)		3	30.00 (0.00–64.56)	
	Smoking/drug/alcohol	8	2.42 (0.75–4.08)		3	1.18 (0.00–2.52)		—	—	—
History of spontaneous abortion	Yes	107	80.45 (73.62–87.28)	<.0001	94	93.07 (88.03–98.11)	<.0001	5	100.00 (100.00–100.00)	—
	No	26	19.55 (12.72–26.38)		7	6.93 (1.89–11.97)		—	—	
Presence of diabetes	Yes	21	6.34 (3.70–8.98)	<.0001	22	8.66 (5.18–12.14)	<.0001	—	—	—
	No	310	93.66 (91.02–96.30)		232	91.34 (87.86–94.82)		10	100.00 (100.00–100.00)	
Presence of hormonal deficiencies (FSH/TSH/etc.)	Yes	30	9.06 (5.95–12.17)	<.0001	29	11.42 (7.48–15.35)	<.0001	3	30.00 (0.00–64.56)	0.2059
	No	301	90.94 (87.83–94.05)		225	88.58 (84.65–92.52)		7	70.00 (35.45–100.00)	
History of congenital disease among first degree relative	Yes	40	12.08 (8.55–15.61)	<.0001	29	11.42 (7.48–15.35)	<.0001	2	20.00 (0.00–50.16)	0.0578
	No	291	87.92 (84.39–91.45)		225	88.58 (84.65–92.52)		8	80.00 (49.84–100.00)	

Table 4.
Descriptive analyses of samples regarding down syndrome.

Variables	Categories	Diagnosed with Turner syndrome					
		Yes			No		
		N	95% CI	P value	N	95% CI	P value
Gender	Male	—	—	—	279	47.77 (43.71–51.84)	<.0001
	Female	11	100.00 (100.00–100.00)		302	51.71 (47.65–55.78)	
Religion	Muslim	4	40.00 (3.06–76.94)	0.5271	148	28.30 (24.43–32.17)	<.0001
	Hindu	6	60.00 (23.06–96.94)		375	71.70 (67.83–75.57)	
History of consanguinity	Yes	—	—	—	28	4.79 (3.06–6.53)	<.0001
	No	11	100.00 (100.00–100.00)		556	95.21 (93.47–96.94)	
Contraceptive used	Yes	2	18.18 (0.00–45.36)	0.0348	102	17.47 (14.38–20.55)	<.0001
	No	9	81.82 (54.64–100.00)		482	82.53 (79.45–85.62)	
Addiction of father	None	5	45.45 (10.37–80.54)	0.5292	336	57.53 (53.51–61.55)	<.0001
	Smoking	4	36.36 (2.47–70.26)		174	29.79 (26.07–33.51)	
	Smoking/ drug	2	18.18 (0.00–45.36)		63	0.79 (8.26–13.31)	
	Smoking/ drug/ alcohol	—	—	—	11	1.88 (0.78–2.99)	
History of spontaneous abortion	Yes	1	50.00 (0.00–100.00)	1.0000	205	86.50 (82.12–90.88)	<.0001
	No	1	50.00 (0.00–100.00)		32	13.50 (9.12–17.88)	
Presence of diabetes	Yes	—	—	—	43	7.36 (5.24–9.49)	<.0001
	No	11	100.00 (100.00–100.00)		541	92.64 (90.51–94.76)	
Presence of hormonal deficiencies (FSH/TSH/ etc.)	Yes	—	—	—	62	10.62 (8.11–13.12)	<.0001
	No	11	100.00 (100.00–100.00)		522	89.38 (86.88–91.89)	
History of congenital disease among first degree relative	Yes	1	9.09 (0.00–29.35)	0.0067	70	11.99 (9.34–14.63)	<.0001
	No	10	90.91 (70.65–100.00)		514	88.01 (85.37–90.66)	

Table 5.
Descriptive analyses of participants regarding turner syndrome (n = 11).

were identified as Down syndrome, 10 (1.68%) as mosaic Down syndrome, while 11 (1.85%) as Turner syndrome, and 11 (1.85%) children with other congenital anomalies.

In **Table 2**: of the total 11 children with congenital abnormalities, five (45.45%) were males. Based on the available information, it was observed that six (75%) belonged to the Hindu religion followed by Muslim (2, 28.52%), one (9.09%) had a history of consanguinity, four (80%) had a history of spontaneous abortion, three (27.27%) reported use of contraceptives, two fathers (18.18%) were addicted to smoking, one (9.09%) was addicted to both smoking and drugs, one subject (9.09%) was diagnosed with diabetes, two subjects (18.18%) with hormonal deficiencies, one subject (9.09%) had a history of congenital disease among first-degree relatives, four (36.36%) were identified as Down syndrome, and none of them with Turner syndrome.

Variables	Categories	Diagnosed as normal (ref = no)	
		Yes	
		OR (95% CI)	P value
Gender (ref = female)	Male	**0.46 (0.33–0.64)**	**<.0001**
Religion (ref = Muslim)	Hindu	1.01 (0.69–1.47)	0.9555
History of consanguinity (ref = no)	Yes	1.08 (0.50–2.31)	0.8449
History of spontaneous abortion (ref = no)	Yes	**0.33 (0.14–0.76)**	**0.0091**
Contraceptives used (ref = no)	Yes	0.76 (0.50–1.16)	0.2084
Addiction of father (ref = none)	Smoking	0.97 (0.67–1.39)	0.8570
	Smoking/drug	0.63 (0.37–1.08)	0.0897
	Smoking/drug/ alcohol	1.55 (0.45–5.38)	0.4928
Presence of diabetes (ref = no)	Yes	0.88 (0.47–1.64)	0.6899
Presence of hormonal deficiencies (FSH/TSH/etc) (ref = no)	Yes	0.80 (0.47–1.36)	0.4067
History of congenital disease among first degree relative (ref = no)	Yes	1.16 (0.70–1.90)	0.5710

Table 6.
Predictors of participants who were diagnosed as normal.

In **Table 3**: of the 283 samples tested to have some genetic abnormalities, 163 (56.79%) were males, 197 (71.38%) belonged to the Hindu religion followed by Muslim (79, 28.62%), 13 (4.53%) had a history of consanguinity, 102 (92.73%) had a history of spontaneous abortion, 56 (19.51%) reported use of contraceptives, 85 fathers (29.62%) were addicted to smoking, 38 (13.24%) to both smoking and drugs, and 4 (1.39%) to either smoking or drugs or alcohol. Among these 283 subjects, 22 (7.67%) were diagnosed with diabetes, 33 (11.50%) had some hormonal deficiencies, and 32 (11.15%) had a history of congenital disease among first-degree relatives.

In **Table 4**: Among the total 254 samples who were diagnosed with Down syndrome, 155 (61.02%) were males, 177 (72.24%) belonged to the Hindu religion followed by Muslim (68, 27.76%), 11 (4.33%) had a history of consanguinity, 94 (93.07%) had a history of spontaneous abortion, 49 (19.29%) couples reported use of contraceptives, 73 (28.74%) fathers were addicted to smoking, 31 (12.20%) to both smoking and drugs and 3 (1.18%) to either smoking or drugs or alcohol, 22 (8.66%) were diagnosed with diabetes, 29 (11.42%) had some hormonal deficiencies, and 29 (11.42%) had a history of congenital disease among first-degree relatives. Among 10 samples who were diagnosed with mosaic Down syndrome, five (50.00%) were males, eight (80%) belonged to the Hindu religion followed by Muslim (2, 20.00%), and two (20.00%) had a history of consanguinity, all had a history of spontaneous abortion, three (30.00%) reported use of contraceptives, four (40.00%) were addicted to smoking, three (30.00%) to both smoking and drugs, while none of them were diagnosed with diabetes, three (30.00%) had some hormonal deficiencies, and two (20.00%) had a history of congenital disease among first-degree relatives.

In **Table 5**: among the total 11 samples who were diagnosed with Turner syndrome and all of them were females, six (60.00%) belonged to the Hindu religion

Variables	Categories	Clinical diagnosed with (ref = neither Down or Mosaic)			
		Down syndrome		Mosaic down syndrome	
		OR (95% CI)	P value	OR (95% CI)	P value
Gender (ref = female)	Male	**2.75 (1.96–3.86)**	**<.0001**	1.76 (0.50–6.19)	0.3809
Religion (ref = Muslim)	Hindu	1.09 (0.74–1.59)	0.6604	1.67 (0.35–8.05)	0.5206
History of consanguinity (ref = no)	Yes	0.95 (0.43–2.11)	0.9069	**5.27 (1.03–26.98)**	**0.0462**
Contraceptives used (ref = no)	Yes	1.28 (0.83–1.97)	0.2567	2.30 (0.58–9.18)	0.2384
Addiction of father (ref = none)	Smoking	0.94 (0.65–1.36)	0.7393	2.52 (0.55–11.49)	0.2319
	Smoking/ drug	1.30 (0.76–2.24)	0.3440	**6.16 (1.19–31.91)**	**0.0302**
	Smoking/ drug/ alcohol	0.49 (0.13–1.87)	0.2945	—	—
History of spontaneous abortion (ref = no)	Yes	**3.26 (1.35–7.86)**	**0.0084**	—	—
Presence of diabetes (ref = no)	Yes	1.40 (0.75–2.61)	0.2890	—	—
Presence of hormonal deficiencies (FSH/TSH/ etc) (ref = no)	Yes	1.29 (0.75–2.22)	0.3497	**4.30 (1.06–17.50)**	**0.0416**
History of congenital disease among first degree relative (ref = no)	Yes	0.94 (0.56–1.56)	0.8042	1.82 (0.37–8.87)	0.4593

Table 7.
Predictors of down syndrome.

followed by Muslim (4, 40.00%) and none had a history of consanguinity. One (50.00%) had a history of spontaneous abortion, two (18.18%) couples reported use of contraceptives, four (36.36%) fathers were addicted to smoking, two (18.18%) to both smoking and drugs, none were diagnosed with diabetes or hormonal deficiencies, and one (9.09%) had a history of congenital disease among first-degree relatives.

In **Table 6**: compared to females, males were 54% (odds ratio, OR = 0.46, 95% CI = 0.33–0.64) less likely to be normal. Additionally, for females who got pregnant and had a history of spontaneous abortion, the chance of being normal was 67% less (odds ratio, OR = 0.33, 95% CI = 0.14–0.76) compared to those who did not have such history.

In **Table 7**: compared to females, males were almost thrice likely (odds ratio, OR = 2.75, 95% CI = 1.96–3.86) to be clinically diagnosed with Down syndrome. Additionally, in females who got pregnant and had a history of spontaneous abortion, the risk of Down syndrome was more than three times higher (odds ratio, OR = 0.33, 95% CI = 0.14–0.76) than those who did not have such history. Subjects with a history of consanguinity had a four times higher risk of being clinically diagnosed with mosaic Down syndrome (odds ratio, OR = 5.27, 95% CI = 1.03–26.98) than those who have no such history. Additionally, history of smoking and drug addiction among fathers was positively (odds ratio, OR = 6.16, 95% CI = 1.19–31.91) associated with a higher likelihood of mosaic Down syndrome than those who did not have such history. Moreover, the risk of being diagnosed with this

Variables	Categories	Diagnosed with Turner syndrome (ref = no)	
		Yes	
		OR (95% CI)	P value
Gender (ref = female)	Male	—	—
Religion (ref = Muslim)	Hindu	0.59 (0.17–2.13)	0.4219
History of consanguinity (ref = no)	Yes	—	—
Contraceptive used (ref = no)	Yes	1.05 (0.22–4.93)	0.9506
Addiction of father (ref = none)	Smoking	1.55 (0.41–5.83)	0.5208
	Smoking/drug	2.13 (0.41–11.24)	0.3715
	Smoking/drug/ alcohol	—	—
History of spontaneous abortion (ref = no)	Yes	0.16 (0.01–2.56)	0.1930
Presence of diabetes (ref = no)	Yes	—	—
Presence of hormonal deficiencies (FSH/TSH/etc.) (ref = no)	Yes	—	—
History of congenital disease among first degree relative (ref = no)	Yes	0.74 (0.09–5.82)	0.7704

Table 8.
Predictors of turner syndrome.

Variables	Categories	Child with congenital abnormalities (ref = no)	
		Yes	
		OR (95% CI)	P value
Gender (ref = female)	Male	0.93 (0.28–3.09)	0.9106
Religion (ref = Muslim)	Hindu	1.20 (0.24–6.01)	0.8245
History of consanguinity (ref = no)	Yes	2.06 (0.26–16.71)	0.4971
Contraceptives used (ref = no)	Yes	1.79 (0.47–6.88)	0.3944
Addiction of father (ref = none)	Smoking	0.47 (0.10–2.25)	0.3470
	Smoking/drug	0.65 (0.08–5.29)	0.6875
	Smoking/drug/ alcohol	—	—
History of spontaneous abortion (ref = no)	Yes	0.63 (0.07–5.85)	0.6875
Presence of diabetes (ref = no)	Yes	1.29 (0.16–10.32)	0.8097
Presence of hormonal deficiencies (FSH/TSH/etc.) (ref = no)	Yes	1.94 (0.41–9.19)	0.4033
History of congenital disease among first degree relative (ref = no)	Yes	0.74 (0.09–5.82)	0.7704

Table 9.
Predictors having congenital abnormalities.

defect was fourfold (odds ratio, OR = 4.30, 95% CI = 1.06–17.50) among participants detected with some hormonal deficiencies than those who did not have such deficiencies.

In **Table 8**: although all the predictors such as male gender, Hindu religion, positive history of consanguinity, history of having the spontaneous abortion, contraceptives use, addiction of father, the presence of diabetes or some hormonal deficiencies and having a history of congenital disease among first-degree relatives seemed to be positively associated with the risk of Turner syndrome, results were not statistically significant due to small sample size and lack of power.

In **Table 9**: the other congenital anomalies did not show any association with the studied factors and results were not statistically significant due to the small sample size and lack of power. Thus, for inconclusive and empirical evidence regarding predictors of participants having a child with congenital abnormalities, a large sample size is required.

4. Discussion

In this study, the different factors such as gender, age, ethnicity, addiction, hormonal status have been analyzed to investigate their possible effect on Down syndrome, Turner syndrome, and other congenital disease prevalence. The distributions of the sample characteristics were significantly different across strata of gender, religion, history of consanguinity, contraceptive used, the addiction of participants' father, whether diagnosed with diabetes or hormonal deficiencies or Down syndrome or Turner syndrome, and history of congenital disease among first-degree relatives and child with congenital abnormalities. The distributions of the children with congenital abnormalities such as ambiguous genitalia or syndactyly were significantly different across strata of history of consanguinity, addiction of parent, whether diagnosed with diabetes or hormonal deficiencies or Down syndrome or Turner syndrome and history of congenital disease among first-degree relatives. Distributions of sample characteristics were significantly different across strata of gender, religion, history of consanguinity, contraceptive used, history of spontaneous abortion, addiction of father, whether diagnosed with diabetes or hormonal deficiencies, and history of congenital disease among first-degree relatives (**Table 3**). The distributions of sample characteristics who were clinically diagnosed with Down syndrome were significantly different across strata of gender, religion, history of consanguinity, contraceptive used, addiction of father, whether diagnosed with diabetes or hormonal deficiencies, and history of congenital disease among first-degree relatives whether individuals diagnosed with mosaic Down syndrome were not significantly different across strata of those factors. Except for the use of contraceptives, distributions of the sample characteristics who were clinically diagnosed with Turner syndrome were not significantly different across the strata of gender, religion, history of consanguinity, addiction of father, whether diagnosed with diabetes or hormonal deficiencies, and history of congenital disease among first-degree relatives. Other predictors, such as Hindu religion, positive history of consanguinity, use of contraceptives, addiction of father, presence of diabetes or hormonal deficiencies, and having a history of congenital disease among first-degree relatives, seemed more likely to be clinically diagnosed as normal but results were not statistically significant due to small sample size and lack of power. Thus, for inconclusive and empirical evidence regarding predictors of clinically normal subjects, a large sample size is required.

On the basis of outcomes, the possible effects of sociodemographic factors are convenient regarding the studied congenital disease occurrence, though a large-scale analysis from all aspects is needed.

5. Conclusion

In this chapter, we have found that some factors such as age, addictions, hormonal imbalances are likely to be associated with Down syndrome, Turner syndrome, and also the other studied congenital diseases. There are several sociodemographic factors that seem to be associated with these congenital disorders, though a large sample size is required for better assessment.

Acknowledgements

We would like to acknowledge all the participants and the analyst team for this work.

Author details

Poulami Majumder[1] and Subrata Kumar Dey[2]*

1 Department of Biotechnology, Maulana Abul Kalam Azad University of Technology, West Bengal, India

2 Swami Vivekananda University, West Bengal, India

*Address all correspondence to: subratadey184@gmail.com

References

[1] Slayton RL, Kantaputra PN. Congenital genetic disorders and syndromes. In: Pediatric Dentistry. 6th ed. Amsterdam: Elsevier; 2019. pp. 244-258.e1. ISBN: 9780323608268

[2] Van Ginderdeuren R, De Vos R, Casteels I, Foets B. Report of a new family with dominant congenital heredity stromal dystrophy of the cornea. Cornea. 2002;**21**(1):118-120

[3] Desai SS. Down syndrome: A review of the literature. Oral Surgery, Oral Medicine, Oral Pathology, Oral Radiology, and Endodontology. 1997; **84**(3):279-285

[4] Bondy CA, Turner Syndrome Consensus Study Group. Care of girls and women with Turner syndrome: A guideline of the Turner Syndrome Study Group. The Journal of Clinical Endocrinology & Metabolism. 2007; **92**(1):10-25

[5] Hoffman JI, Kaplan S. The incidence of congenital heart disease. Journal of the American College of Cardiology. 2002;**39**(12):1890-1900

[6] Fraser FC. The genetics of cleft lip and cleft palate. American Journal of Human Genetics. 1970;**22**(3):336

[7] Hallmayer J, Cleveland S, Torres A, Phillips J, Cohen B, Torigoe T, et al. Genetic heritability and shared environmental factors among twin pairs with autism. Archives of General Psychiatry. 2011;**68**(11):1095-1102

[8] Liu F, Yang YN, Xie X, Li XM, Ma X, Fu ZY, et al. Prevalence of congenital heart disease in Xinjiang multi-ethnic region of China. PLoS One. 2015;**10**(8):e0133961

[9] De Silva APGS, Thattil RO, Samita S. Estimation of food and nutrition factor in human development. Tropical Agricultural Research. 2000;**12**:287-296

[10] Egbe A, Uppu S, Stroustrup A, Lee S, Ho D, Srivastava S. Incidences and sociodemographics of specific congenital heart diseases in the United States of America: an evaluation of hospital discharge diagnoses. Pediatric Cardiology. 2014;**35**(6):975-982

[11] Majumder P, Bhaumik P, Ghosh P, Bhattacharya M, Ghosh S, Dey SK. Recent advances in research on Down syndrome. Health Problems in Down Syndrome. 2015:87. DOI: 10.5772/60648

[12] Bhattacharya M, Bhaumik P, Ghosh P, Majumder P, Kumar Dey S. telomere length inheritance and shortening in trisomy 21. Fetal and Pediatric Pathology. 2020;**39**(5): 390-400

[13] Ghosh S, Hong CS, Feingold E, Ghosh P, Ghosh P, Bhaumik P, et al. Epidemiology of Down syndrome: New insight into the multidimensional interactions among genetic and environmental risk factors in the oocyte. American Journal of Epidemiology. 2011;**174**(9):1009-1016

[14] Ghosh S, Bhaumik P, Ghosh P, Dey SK. Chromosome 21 non-disjunction and Down syndrome birth in an Indian cohort: Analysis of incidence and aetiology from family linkage data. Genetics Research. 2010; **92**(3):189-197

[15] Majumder P, Ghosh S, Dey SK. Spontaneous abortion of aneuploidy foetus enhances the risk of Down syndrome birth: Implication of epidemiological factors. International Journal of Current Biotechnology (IJCB). 2014;**2**(12):9-15. ISSN-2321-8371

[16] Zagon IS, Slotkin TA, editors. Maternal Substance Abuse and the Developing Nervous System. San Diego, California: Academic Press; 2012

[17] Niccols A. Fetal alcohol syndrome and the developing socio-emotional brain. Brain and Cognition. 2007;**65**(1): 135-142

[18] Saenger P, Wikland KA, Conway GS, Davenport M, Gravholt CH, Hintz R, et al. Recommendations for the diagnosis and management of Turner syndrome. The Journal of Clinical Endocrinology & Metabolism. 2001;**86**(7):3061-3069

[19] Mamula CJ, Erhard RE, Piva SR. Cervical radiculopathy or Parsonage-Turner syndrome: Differential diagnosis of a patient with neck and upper extremity symptoms. Journal of Orthopaedic & Sports Physical Therapy. 2005;**35**(10):659-664

[20] Silva ALD, Lima RL, Ribeiro LA, Moretti-Ferreira D. X monosomy and balanced Robertsonian translocation in a girl with Turner Syndrome. Genetics and Molecular Biology. 2006;**29**:47-48

[21] Soares S, Templado C, Blanco J, Egozcue J, Vidal F. Numerical chromosome abnormalities in the spermatozoa of the fathers of children with trisomy 21 of paternal origin: Generalised tendency to meiotic non-disjunction. Human Genetics. 2001; **108**(2):134-139

[22] Leslie EJ, Marazita ML. Genetics of cleft lip and cleft palate. American Journal of Medical Genetics Part C: Seminars in Medical Genetics. 2013; **163**(4):246-258

[23] Sommerlad BC. A technique for cleft palate repair. Plastic and Reconstructive Surgery. 2003;**112**(6): 1542-1548

[24] Larossa D. The state of the art in cleft palate surgery. The Cleft Palate-Craniofacial Journal. 2000;**37**(3): 225-228

[25] Wermker K, Lünenbürger H, Joos U, Kleinheinz J, Jung S. Results of speech improvement following simultaneous push-back together with velopharyngeal flap surgery in cleft palate patients. Journal of Cranio-Maxillofacial Surgery. 2014;**42**(5): 525-530

[26] Scherer NJ, D'Antonio LL, McGahey H. Early intervention for speech impairment in children with cleft palate. The Cleft Palate-Craniofacial Journal. 2008;**45**(1):18-31

[27] Malik S. Syndactyly: Phenotypes, genetics and current classification. European Journal of Human Genetics. 2012;**20**(8):817-824

[28] Ahmed SF, Rodie M. Investigation and initial management of ambiguous genitalia. Best Practice & Research Clinical Endocrinology & Metabolism. 2010;**24**(2):197-218

[29] Göllü G, Yıldız RV, Bingol-Kologlu M, Yagmurlu A, Senyücel MF, Aktug T, et al. Ambiguous genitalia: An overview of 17 years' experience. Journal of Pediatric Surgery. 2007;**42**(5):840-844

[30] Koebnick C, Langer-Gould AM, Gould MK, Chao CR, Iyer RL, Smith N, et al. Sociodemographic characteristics of members of a large, integrated health care system: Comparison with US Census Bureau data. The Permanente Journal. 2012;**16**(3):37

Chapter 5

What Causes Down Syndrome?

Emine Ikbal Atli

Abstract

Trisomy 21 (Down Syndrome) is the model human phenotype for all genome gain-dosage imbalance situations, including microduplications. Years after the sequencing of chromosome 21, the discovery of functional genomics and the creation of multiple cellular and mouse models provided an unprecedented opportunity to demonstrate the molecular consequences of genome dosage imbalance. It was stated years ago that Down syndrome, caused by meiotic separation of chromosome 21 in humans, is associated with advanced maternal age, but defining and understanding other risk factors is insufficient. Commonly referred to as Down syndrome (DS) in humans, trisomy 21 is the most cited genetic cause of mental retardation. In about 95% of cases, the extra chromosome occurs as a result of meiotic non- nondisjunction (NDJ) or abnormal separation of chromosomes. In most of these cases the error occurs during maternal oogenesis, especially in meiosis I.

Keywords: trisomy 21, chromosome 21, non- nondisjunction, down syndrome, genetics

1. Introduction

More than 50 years have passed since trisomy 21 was identified as the cause of Down syndrome. After that date, the first link between a clinical disorder and a chromosomal abnormality was established. In the intervening half century, the importance of numerical chromosome abnormalities for human disease pathology has been well established.

Studies with live births in the 1960s and 1970s showed that about 0,3% of newborns were trisomic or monosomic, while subsequent studies of spontaneous abortions found a much higher incidence of about 35%. Taken together, these studies revealed aneuploidy as the leading known cause of congenital birth defects and miscarriages, showing that most cases of aneuploidy disappear in utero [1–3].

In humans, trisomy 21, commonly referred to as Down syndrome (DS), is the most common genetic cause of mental retardation. In about 95% of cases, the excess chromosome occurs as a result of meiotic nondisjunction (NDJ) or incorrect dissociation of chromosomes [4, 5]. In most of the cases, the error occurs during maternal oogenesis, especially in meiosis I (MI) [6]. Advanced maternal age and defective recombination are two risk factors that have been reported to be associated with DS for cases where extra chromosome arises in the oocyte. The process of oogenesis is long and is a cycle that involves meiotic arrest, making it more vulnerable to improper assembly of chromosomes than spermatogenesis. Also, with increasing age, there is a rapid degradation of spindle thread formation in sister chromatid cohesion or anaphase separation of sister chromatids in oocytes, and this poses the risk of NDJ in both MI and MII [7–11].

Through recombinant DNA technology, a new technique has become available to study the origin and mechanisms of chromosomal abnormalities using DNA polymorphism analysis. Initially, such analyzes used chromosome 21-specific DNA probes to detect restriction fragment length polymorphisms. The development of the polymerase chain reaction (PCR) amplification technique has enabled the identification of new and highly informative classes of DNA polymorphisms (microsatellites or simple sequence repeat (SSR) polymorphisms) in the human genome. In particular, multi-allelic and easily typeable micro satellites have contributed to chromosomal nondisjunction studies in recent years [12–14].

Meiotic meiosis I or II examination of nondisjunction in trisomy 21 by DNA polymorphism analysis could not be performed due to the absence of centromeric markers. Alphaid DNA polymorphisms specific to the human chromosome 21 centromere were identified years ago, but these markers were unlikely to provide information on the process and were not useful for routine nondisjunction studies. However, alfoid DNA polymorphisms were localized in the genetic linkage map of chromosome 21(**Figure 1**), and an estimate of the genetic distance between the centromere and the closest pericentromeric markers on the long arm of chromosome 21 was made [4, 9, 16].

Two large collaborative studies used DNA polymorphism involving the long arm of human chromosome 21 to determine the parental origin of separation in trisomy 21. Such studies estimate that only 5% of trisomy 21 (of a total of 304 families studied) originates from the father and attributes the difference in cytogenetic studies to the increased accuracy of DNA polymorphism analysis as shown by inaccurate

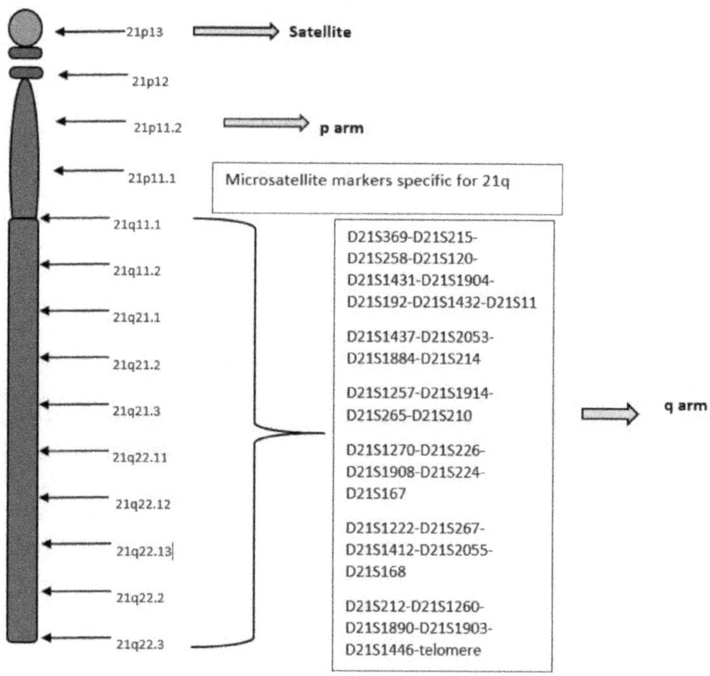

Figure 1.
Short tandem repeat (STR) markers used to infer the origin of the meiotic error and characterization of the recombination profile [15].

cytogenetic determinations in a subgroup of families. Other population-based studies show paternal meiotic errors in the 5–9% range [17, 18].

For example, the absence of detectable recombination or just a single telomeric change may be associated with MI NDJ errors, and this pattern is more common in the younger maternal age group than in the older maternal group. In contrast, it shows that MII errors are clearly associated with pericentromeric changes in older maternal age groups [19].

A molecular study found high differences in mean maternal ages between maternal origin cases and paternal origin cases. This demonstrated that the maternal age effect in Down syndrome is limited to maternal nondisjunction and does not provide evidence for a comfortable selection against trisomic fetuses in older women [20, 21].

2. Sex-specific differences in meiosis

As discussed in many studies, studies of clinically recognized pregnancies indicate that most human aneuploidy is of maternal origin. The question then arises: why is female meiosis so prone to error? In this section, we review oocyte development and summarize the latest evidence that errors in the oocyte that predispose to chromosome misgrouping are increased, and that gender-specific differences in meiotic cell cycle checkpoints allow oocytes with these errors to develop into mature eggs [3, 22].

In mammals, meiotic recombination occurs in the fetal ovary and the significance of the resulting physical connections for chromosome separation has been well observed. Studies in the 1990s identified transitions that could not be recombined and / or optimally positioned as significant contributors to human trisomy.

Changing recombination is essential here. It is related to mother-derived trisomies as well as those originating from the father. However, the female is clearly at greater risk, as most aneuploidy occurs during oogenesis. Therefore, either more recombination errors are made in the female or these errors are removed more efficiently in the male [23, 24].

The immunofluorescence methodology has made it possible to examine cross-linked proteins in pachytene spermatocytes and oocytes and thus test these alternatives. Interestingly, almost all chromosomes in males are joined by at least one crossover, but the same is not true for females [4, 14, 18].

Studies have shown that; The conclusion is that more than 10% of all human oocytes contain at least one "non-crossing" bivalent. Since half of all these divalent ones are expected to result in aneuploidy (**Figure 2**), the stage seems to have been adjusted for meiotic errors from the onset of oogenesis.

As suggested based on cytogenetic studies with no evidence of a difference in mean maternal age between maternal and paternal trisomy 21 cases. A factor associated with aging of the oocyte therefore appears to be responsible for the maternal age effect in Down syndrome.

Among maternal errors, approximately 75% are considered errors in meiosis I and 25% as errors in meiosis II. Maternal meiosis I and II errors are linked to increased maternal age [25–27]. Two studies of cytogenetic short-arm heteromorphisms and microsatellite DNA polymorphisms showed inconsistencies regarding the meiotic period of non-separation and suggested pericentromeric increased recombination associated with nondisjunction. The place where chiasma occurs is the middle of the chromosome arm and then recombination is necessary for proper

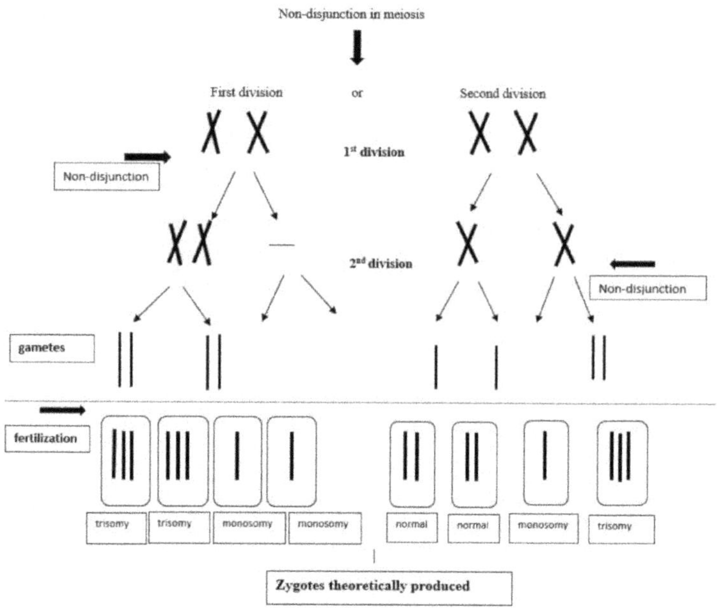

Figure 2.
Homogeneous due to meiotic non-disjunction.

chromosome separation as it holds the chromatids tightly and balances the attraction to opposite poles [28, 29].

Meiotic recombination was thought to stabilize matched homologs to ensure their proper separation. However, the process is stochastic and may not be handled properly even in euploid samples. Thus, achiasmate chromosomes are vulnerable to malsegregation and this condition gradually increases with age due to the rapid degradation of the protein mechanism within oocytes responsible for surveillance and separation of chromosomes. A chiasma located near the telomere of the chromosome probably attaches the homolog to the spindle weaklier due to loss of cohesion and directs the kinetochore precisely towards the opposite pole. On the other hand, chiasmata close to the center occurs during MI, which causes chromosome entanglement so the bivalent cannot be separated correctly. In this way the MII can pass into the anaphase plate and then result in the reduction section; as a result, a disomic gamete is produced [30, 31].

Epidemiological studies have identified some environmental, habitual and socio-economic factors that may pose a risk for Ch21 NDJ. These can be observed in both MI and MII errors depending on maternal age or independent of maternal age. When we consider these findings, it is clear that Ch21 NDJ risk is a multifactorial event that interacts with genetic and environmental factors.

About 5% of trisomy 21 cases are likely due to the mitotic (postzygotic) non-disjunction of chromosome 21 in the early embryo. This was demonstrated by the identification of pericentromeric DNA markers and the lack of recombination observed along the entire long arm of chromosome 21. Mitotic errors are not associated with advanced maternal age and do not show any preference depending on the parental origin of the replica chromosome 21. Mosaic with a normal cell line occurs in about 2–4% of newborns with Down syndrome. By DNA polymorphism analysis performed in 17 families with mosaic trisomy 21 probands, it showed that most cases were caused by a trisomic zygote with mitotic loss of one chromosome (**Table 1**) [32, 33].

Origin	Number of cases	%	Meiotic recombination
Maternal	732	90,7	
MI	556	68,9	Reduced
MII	176	21,8	Increased
Paternal	44	5,5	
MI	17	2,1	Reduced
MII	27	3,3	
Mitotic	31	3,8	
Maternal	17	2,1	
Paternal	14	1,7	

MI: Meosis I, MII: Meosis II, Maternal and Paternal refer to parental origin of the chromosome that was duplicated by postzygotic nondisjunction

Table 1.
Origin of nondisjunction in human trisomy 21 by DNA polymorphism analysis [31, 33–35].

3. Changes in recombination

Failure to nondisjunction in maternal meiosis I is associated with reduced recombination between unallocated chromosomes 21, suggesting an important role for pairing / recombination errors or reduced recombination in the etiology of trisomy 21. Subsequent results showed an overall reduction in recombination, but with increased recombination in the distant region of 21q.

Meiotic outcome group	Maternal age group	Number of observed events	Frequency of observed number recombinants			Frequency of the number inferred exchanges		
			0	1	≥2	0	1	≥2
MI								
	Young (<29 yrs)	175	0,70	0,20	0,10	0,47	0,32	0,21
	Mid (29–34 yrs)	197	0,56	0,35	0,10	0,18	0,64	0,19
	Old (>34 yrs)	243	0,64	0,27	0,09	0,27	0,49	0,24
MII								
	Young (<29 yrs)	58	—	0,66	0,34	—	0,22	0,78
	Mid (29–34 yrs)	69	—	0,78	0,22	—	0,51	0,49
	Old (>34 yrs)	126	—	0,81	0,19	—	0,57	0,44
Euploid								
	All Ages	152	0,52	0,39	0,09	0,20	0,50	0,30

Table 2.
Frequency distribution of observed recombinants and inferred exchanges for each meiotic outcome group stratified by maternal age group [10].

Unpredictably, nondisjunction in meiosis II is due to the increased recombination occurring in meiosis I suggesting that all errors are due to meiosis I. The recombination rate remains constant with advancing maternal age. However, possible chiasmate configurations of chromosome 21 appear more susceptible to nondisjunction in older oocytes than younger oocytes (**Table 2**).

Analysis of the chiasma configuration showed that the failure of a proximal recombination (or the presence of a telomeric recombination) tends to be nondisjunction in meiosis I, while the presence of pericentromeric change appears to be nondisjunction in meiosis II [30, 31, 36, 37].

These findings are very effective in understanding the etiology of trisomy 21 and may explain why both maternal meiosis I and II errors are associated with increased maternal age. A two-hit nondisjunction model has been proposed where the first hit is the prenatal establishment of a sensitive tetrad and the second hit is the disruption of a meiotic process that increases the risk of nondisjunction of the susceptible configuration. The second hit can involve any element of the meiotic process and can be the basis for the maternal age effect. Recent studies have found signs indicating a reduction in the recombination rate in the total genome of eggs with chromosome 21 nondisjoined, meaning that the reduction in recombination is not limited to nondisjoined chromosomes but extends to other chromosomes as well [22].

The two-beat non-separation model needs to be validated with further study from other chromosomes and direct observation with oocytes.

4. Paternal nondisjunction

In the paternal nondisjunction of chromosome 21, there is mainly meiosis II error, as DNA polymorphisms show, in contrast to meiosis I errors and maternal nondisjunction.

Therefore, the mechanisms associated with paternal nondisjunction will likely differ from those associated with maternal nondisjunction.

In live births with Down syndrome; there is a well-known increasing ratio (about 1.15) between the sexes. This effect is limited to free trisomy 21 cases and does not include translocation-style trisomies, suggesting that increased sex ratio is associated with free trisomy 21 per se, not gender-based differential selection. As a result of molecular studies, it has been revealed that among the meiotic errors of the father, a rather high sex ratio (3.50) and male proband excess, in contrast to paternal mitotic errors and maternal errors, are specific to MII errors.

As with maternal meiosis, there is reduced recombination across the nondisjoined 21. chromosome involved in the 22 paternal nondisjunction cases, but there is no difference in recombination between the 27 paternal MII cases compared to controls [14, 18, 34].

5. Recurrence risk of nondisjunction

Two molecular studies with families with free trisomy 21 relapse showed that mosaicism in parents is an important etiological factor and that this possibility alone may explain recurrent trisomy 21 in most families. In only a small number of families, the possibility of genetic predisposition for chromosomal nondisjunction could not be excluded [32, 35].

It has been previously shown that live born children with free trisomy 21 for chromosomally normal parents whose maternal age is less than 30 years have a significantly increased risk of recurrence [35].

6. Risk factors

Many factors have been suggested as risk factors for nondisjunction in the past, but only in the last few studies identified the source of nondisjunction by DNA analysis. The increased frequency of the apolipoprotein E (APOE) allele Â4 was more observed in young mothers with MII errors in a population-scale study of Down syndrome in Denmark. This finding showed an increased risk of Alzheimer's disease in a subgroup of young Down syndrome mothers and suggested the APOE E4 allele as a risk factor for nondisjunction in young mothers [36–38].

An association between an intron polymorphism in the presenilin-1 gene and maternal MII errors was identified in the same population-based study and the function of presenilin proteins in chromosome segregation was determined and thought to be related to subcellular localization.

Another population-based study revealed an association with young MII mothers and maternal smoking and oral contraceptive use.

Both studies have found an association in young MII mothers, and the proposed risk factors support the ovarian risky microcirculation hypothesis to explain the effect of maternal age on nondisjunction, and it should not be overlooked.

Oocytes from hypoxic follicles under heavy exposure showed abnormalities in the organization of chromosomes on the metaphase spindle at high frequencies.

When we look at the two hit nondisjunction model, the findings suggest that aging alone is sufficient to disrupt the meiosis process, but there is a higher requirement for a genetic or environmental factor for nondisjunction to occur in young women.

A different recent study showed abnormal folate metabolism in mothers with Down syndrome; It was reported that the C677T mutation in the methylenetetrahydrofolate reductase (MTHFR) gene was higher in mothers with Down syndrome than in control mothers. However, the study included a small number of mothers and was not population-based, and so the source of nondisjunction could not be determined. Nevertheless, the study may support the at-risk microcirculation hypothesis as hyperhomocysteinemia is a known risk factor for vascular disease and the common MTHFR C677T mutation in the homozygous state is associated with mild hyperhomocysteinemia [39–42].

7. Conclusions

As a result, it shows that there is a high frequency of chromosome abnormalities throughout embryonic development as a result of accumulated errors during gametogenesis and early mitotic divisions. Advancing female age is associated with increased rates of aneuploidy in oocytes and embryos. Especially during female meiosis, excessive chromosome losses, anaphase delay of chromosomes and / or capturing of the spindle by microtubules (congression failure) are important mechanisms that cause aneuploidy during oogenesis and continue to have a significant effect during the first few mitotic divisions. Studies of abortions and molecular genetic analyzes of chromosomal abnormalities revealed that most aneuploidies occur during female meiosis, usually as a result of splitting in the first meiotic division. Aneuploidies and, to a lesser extent, male-meiotic errors due to both premature separation of sister chromatids during female meiotic divisions and mitotic chromosome malsegregation are quite common. The fact that aneuploidies caused by these disturbances are rarely seen later in pregnancy increases the likelihood that the origin of aneuploidy may somehow affect the impact on embryo viability.

While interest in the development and refinement of culture systems to support the development of functional gametes from stem cells for the treatment of infertility has been intense, so far those working in these areas have shown little interest in the meiotic process. Obviously, the successful production of normal gametes in vitro will require great attention to meiotic details and a full understanding of the differences between the sexes.

Acknowledgements

Thanks to everyone to IntechOpen publishing team and Author Service Manager.

Conflict of interest

The authors declare no conflict of interest.

Acronyms and abbreviations

DS	Down syndrome
NDJ	Non- nondisjunction
MI	Meiosis I
MII	Meiosis II
PCR	Polymerase chain reaction
SSR	Microsatellites or simple sequence repeat
STR	Short tandem repeat
APOE	Apolipoprotein E
MTHFR	Methylenetetrahydrofolate reductase.

Author details

Emine Ikbal Atli
Faculty of Medicine, Department of Medical Genetics, Edirne, Trakya University, Edirne, Turkey

*Address all correspondence to: eikbalatli@trakya.edu.tr

References

[1] Lejeune J , Turpin R, Gautier M. Mongolism; a chromosomal disease (trisomy). Bull. Acad. Natl Med. 1959; 143:256-265. [PubMed: 13662687]

[2] Jacobs PA, Baikie AG, Court Brown WM, Strong JA. The somatic chromosomes in mongolism. Lancet. 1959; 1:710. [PubMed: 13642857]

[3] Hassold T, Hunt P. To err (meiotically) is human: the genesis of human aneuploidy. Nature Rev. Genet. 2001; 2:280-291. [PubMed: 11283700

[4] Antonarakis SE. Parental origin of the extra chromosome in trisomy 21 as indicated by analysis of DNA polymorphisms. Down Syndrome Collaborative Group. N Engl J Med. 1991; 324:872-876. [PubMed: 1825697]

[5] Freeman SB, Allen EG, Oxford-Wright CL, Tinker SW, Druschel C, Hobbs CA, O'Leary LA, Romitti PA, Royle MH, Torfs CP, Sherman SL. The National Down Syndrome Project: Design and implementation. Public Health Rep. 2007; 122:62-72. [PubMed: 17236610]

[6] Sherman SL, Allen EG, Bean L, Freeman SB. Epidemiology of Down Syndrome. Mental Retard And Dev Disab. 2007; 13:221-227.

[7] Hassold T, Chiu D. Maternal age specific rate of numerical chromosome anomalies with special reference to trisomy. Hum Genet. 1985; 70:11-17. [PubMed: 3997148]

[8] Warren AC, Chakravarti A, Wong C, Slaugenhaupt SA, Halloran SL, Watkins PC, Metaxotou C, Antonarakis SE. Evidence for reduced recombination on the nondisjoined chromosomes 21 in Down syndrome. Science. 1987; 237:652-654. [PubMed: 2955519]

[9] Sherman SL, Takaesu N, Freeman SB, Grantham M, Phillips C, Blackstone RD, Jacobs PA, Cockwell AE, Freeman V, Uchida I, Mikkelsen M, Kurnit DM, Buraczynska M, Keats BJB, Hassold TJ. Trisomy 21: association between reduced recombination and nondisjunction. Am J Hum Genet. 1991; 49:608-620. [PubMed: 1831960]

[10] Oliver TR, Feingold E, Yu K, Cheung V, Tinker S, Yadav-Shah M, Masse N, Sherman SL. New insight into Human Nondisjunction of Chromosome 21 in Oocyte. PloS Genet. 2008; 4(3): e1000033. [PubMed: 18369452]

[11] Wolstenholme J, Angell RR. Maternal age and trisomy--a unifying mechanism of formation. Chromosoma. 2000; 109:435-438. [PubMed: 11151672]

[12] Weber JL, May PE: Abundant class of human DNA polymorphisms which can be typed using the polymerase chain reaction. Am J hum Genet 44:388-396 (1989).

[13] Economou EP, Bergen AW, Warren AC, Antonarakis SE: The polydeoxyadenylate tract of Alu repetitive elements is polymorphic in the human genome. Proc natl Acad Sci, USA 87:2951-2954 (1990).

[14] Petersen MB, Mikkelsen M. Nondisjunction in trisomy 21: origin and mechanisms. Cytogenet Cell Genet. 2000;91(1-4):199-203. doi: 10.1159/000056844. PMID: 11173856.

[15] Ray A, Oliver TR, Halder P, Pal U, Sarkar S, Dutta S, Ghosh S. Risk of Down syndrome birth: Consanguineous marriage is associated with maternal meiosis-II nondisjunction at younger age and without any detectable recombination error. Am J Med Genet A. 2018 Nov;176(11):2342-2349. doi: 10.1002/ajmg.a.40511. Epub 2018 Sep 21. PMID: 30240118.

[16] Jabs EW, Warren AC, Taylor EW, Colyer CR, Meyers DA, Antonarakis SE: Alphoid DNA polymorphisms for chromosome 21 can be distinguished from those of chromosome 13 using probes homologous to both. Genomics 9:141-146 (1991).

[17] Lorber BJ, Grantham M, Peters J, Willard HF, Hassold TJ: Nondisjunction of chromosome 21: comparisons of cytogenetic and molecular studies of the meiotic stage and parent of origin. Am J hum Genet 51:1265-1276 (1992).

[18] Petersen MB, Frantzen M, Antonarakis SE, Warren AC, Van Broeckhoven C, Chakravarti A, Cox TK, Lund C, Olsen B, Poulsen H, Sand A, Tommerup N, Mikkelsen M: Comparative study of microsatellite and cytogenetic markers for detecting the origin of the nondisjoined chromosome 21 in Down syndrome. Am J hum Genet 51:516-525 (1992).

[19] Cheung, V. G., Burdick, J. T., Hirschmann, D., & Morley, M. (2007). Polymorphic variation in human meiotic recombination. American Journal of Human Genetics, 80, 526-530.

[20] Ghosh, S., Ghosh, P., & Dey, S. K. (2014). Altered incidence of meiotic errors and Down syndrome birth under extreme low socioeconomic exposure in the Sundarban area of India. Journal of Community Genetics, 5, 119-124.

[21] Ghosh, S., Hong, C.S., Feingold, E., Ghosh, P., Ghosh, P., Bhaumik,P. & Dey, S.K. (2011).Epidemiology of Down syndrome: New insight into the multidimensional interactions among genetic and environmental risk factors in the oocyte. American Journal of Epidemiology, 174,1009-1016.

[22] Nagaoka SI, Hassold TJ, Hunt PA. Human aneuploidy: mechanisms and new insights into an age-old problem. Nat Rev Genet. 2012 Jun 18;13(7):493-504. doi: 10.1038/nrg3245. PMID: 22705668; PMCID: PMC3551553.

[23] Lynn A, et al. Covariation of synaptonemal complex length and mammalian meiotic exchange rates. Science. 2002; 296:2222-2225. [PubMed: 12052900]

[24] Cheng EY, et al. Meiotic recombination in human oocytes. PLoS Genet. 2009; 5:e1000661. [PubMed: 19763179] This is a study of human fetal oocytes that provides evidence that recombination errors occurring during fetal development set the stage for nondisjunction in the adult

[25] Baudat F, et al. PRDM9 is a major determinant of meiotic recombination hotspots in humans and mice. Science. 2010; 327:836-840. [PubMed: 20044539]

[26] Kong A, et al. Sequence variants in the RNF212 gene associate with genome-wide recombination rate. Science. 2008; 319:1398-1401. [PubMed: 18239089]

[27] Lynn A, Ashley T, Hassold T. Variation in human meiotic recombination. Annu. Rev. Genom. Hum. Genet. 2004; 5:317-349.

[28] Mikkelsen M, Hallberg A, Poulsen H, Frantzen M, Hansen J, Petersen MB: Epidemiological study of Down's syndrome in Denmark, including family studies of chromosomes and DNA markers. Dev Brain Dysfunct 8:4-12 (1995).

[29] Yoon PW, Freeman SB, Sherman SL, Taft LF, Gu Y, Pettay D, Dana Flanders W, Khoury MJ, Hassold TJ: Advanced maternal age and the risk of Down syndrome characterized by the meiotic stage of the chromosomal error: a population-based study. Am J hum Genet 58:628-633 (1996).

[30] Lamb NE, Feingold E, Savage A, Avramopoulos D, Freeman S, Gu Y,

Hallberg A, Hersey J, Karadima G, Pettay D, Saker D, Shen J, Taft L, Mikkelsen M, Petersen MB, Hassold T, Sherman SL: Characterization of susceptible chiasma configurations that increase the risk for maternal nondisjunction of chromosome 21. Hum molec Genet 6:1391-1399 (1997).

[31] Lamb NE, Freeman SB, Savage-Austin A, Pettay D, Taft L, Hersey J, Gu Y, Shen J, Saker D, May KM, Avramopoulos D, Petersen MB, Hallberg A, Mikkelsen M, Hassold TJ, Sherman SL: Susceptible chiasmate configurations of chromosome 21 predispose to non-disjunction in both maternal meiosis I and meiosis II errors. Nature Genet 14:400-405 (1996)

[32] Pangalos C, Avramopoulos D, Blouin J-L, Raoul O, deBlois M-C, Prieur M, Schinzel AA, Gika M, Abazis D, Antonarakis SE: Understanding the mechanism(s) of mosaic trisomy 21 by using DNA polymorphism analysis. Am J hum Genet 54:473-481 (1994).

[33] Antonarakis SE, Avramopoulos D, Blouin J-L, Talbot CC Jr, Schinzel AA: Mitotic errors in somatic cells cause trisomy 21 in about 4.5% of cases and are not associated with advanced maternal age. Nature Genet 3:146-150 (1993).

[34] Savage AR, Petersen MB, Pettay D, Taft L, Allran K, Freeman SB, Karadima G, Avramopoulos D, Torfs C, Mikkelsen M, Hassold TJ, Sherman SL: Elucidating the mechanisms of paternal non-disjunction of chromosome 21 in humans. Hum molec Genet 7:1221-1227 (1998).

[35] James SJ, Pogribna M, Pogribny IP, Melnyk S, Hihe RJ, Gibson JB, Yi P, Tafoya DL, Swenson DH, Wilson VL, Gaylor DW: Abnormal folate metabolism and mutation in the methylenetetrahydrofolate reductase gene may be maternal risk factors for Down syndrome. Am J Clin Nutr 70:495-501 (1999).

[36] Savage Brown A, Feingold E, Brown KW, Sherman SL: Genome-wide variation in recombination in female meiosis: a risk factor for non-disjunction of chromosome 21. Hum molec Genet 9:515-523 (2000).

[37] Angell R: First-meiotic-division nondisjunction in human oocytes. Am J Hum Genet 61:23-32 (1997).

[38] Li J, Xu M, Zhou H, Ma J, Potter H: Alzheimer presenilins in the nuclear membrane, interphase kinetochores, and centrosomes suggest a role in chromosome segregation. Cell 90:917-927 (1997).

[39] Warburton D: Invited editorial. Human female meiosis: new insights into an error-prone process. Am Jhum Genet 61:1-4 (1997).

[40] Yang Q, Sherman SL, Hassold TJ, Allran K, Taft L, Pettay D, Khoury MJ, Erickson JD, Freeman SB: Risk factors for trisomy 21: maternal cigarette smoking and oral contraceptive use in a population-based case-control study. Genetics in Medicine 1:80-88 (1999)

[41] Avramopoulos D, Mikkelsen M, Vassilopoulos D, Grigoriadou M, Petersen MB: Apolipoprotein E allele distribution in parents of Down's syndrome children. Lancet 347:862-865 (1996).

[42] Van Blerkom J, Antczak M, Schrader R: The developmental potential of the human oocyte is related to the dissolved oxygen content of follicular fluid: association with vascular endothelial growth factor levels and perifollicular blood flow characteristics. Hum Reprod 12:1047-1055 (1997).

Chapter 6

Phenotypes Associated with Down Syndrome and Causative Genes

Fatma Söylemez

Abstract

Down syndrome (DS) is the most common chromosomal condition associated with mental retardation and is characterized by a variety of additional clinical findings. It occurs in approximately 1 of 800 births worldwide. DS is associated with number of phenotypes including heart defects, leukemia, Alzheimer's disease, hypertension etc. Individuals with DS are affected by these diseases to variable rates, so understanding the reason for this variation is an important challenge. Multiple genes located both on chromosome 21 and other regions of the genome such as the polymorphism of the amyloid precursor protein (APP) gene contribute to clinical variations. Information on these genetic variations allows early diagnosis and treatment of phenotypes associated with DS. In this chapter, an overview of disease management will be provided by reviewing the genes or miRNAs that cause DS-associated phenotypes.

Keywords: Down syndrome, disease, phenotypes, genes, variation

1. Introduction

Down syndrome is one of the best-recognized and most common chromosome disorders caused by the presence of a third copy of chromosome 21 (Trisomy 21). It is the most common genetic cause of mental retardation. The incidence of Down syndrome is approximately 1/800 newborns [1, 2]. The risk for having a child with Down syndrome increases with maternal age. There are several features that occur in the entire DS population, including learning disability, craniofacial abnormality, and hypotonia [3]. In addition to learning difficulties, Down syndrome patients face a variety of health problems, including congenital heart disease, Alzheimer's diseases (AD), leukemia, cancers and gastrointestinal defects. The 200 to 300 genes on chromosome 21 have been identified as causatives to clinical features of the syndrome. Multiple genes such as polymorphisms of the Down syndrome cell adhesion molecule (DSCAM) and APP gene, both on chromosome 21 and other regions of the genome, are known to contribute to variation in clinical manifestations [4].

2. Down syndrome genetics and typical features

The most common reason for having a baby with DS is the presence of an extra copy of chromosome 21 that results in trisomy. Trisomy 21 (47,XX,+ 21 or 47,XY,+ 21) is caused by a failure of the chromosome 21 to separate during egg or sperm development (**Figure 1**). The other causes can be Robertsonian translocation and isochromosomal or ring chromosome [5]. Robertsonian translocation occurs in only 2–4%

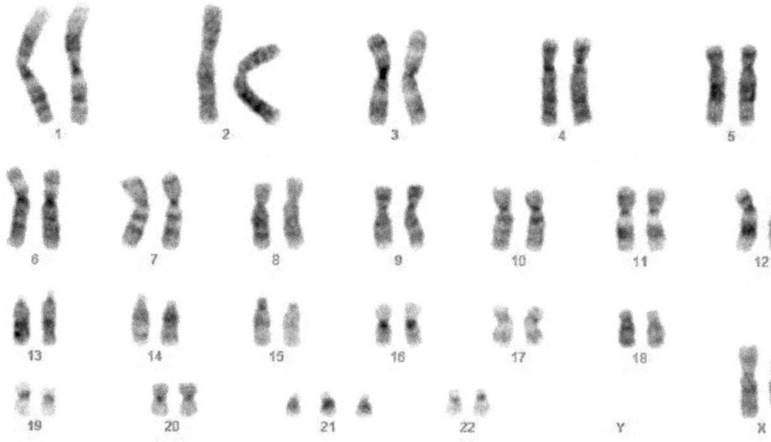

Figure 1.
47,XX,+21. Down syndrome karyotype demonstrating trisomy 21 (female) (Karyotype prepared by Fatma Soylemez).

of cases and occurs when the long arm of the 21st chromosome is attached to another submetacentric chromosome. Mosaicism occurs as a result of an error in cell division or a false division after fertilization. This is why people with mosaic DS have two cell lines in their tissues, one containing a normal number of chromosomes and the other an extra chromosome 21 [5]. Mosaicism of trisomy 21 and partial trisomy 21 are other genetic diagnoses and are usually associated with fewer clinical features of DS. Trisomy 21 and partial trisomy 21 mosaicism are generally associated with less clinical features of DS [4].

DS has high genetic complexity and phenotype variability [6, 7]. DS individual has some physical characteristics like a small chin, slanted eye, poor muscle tone, a flat nasal bridge, a single crease of the palm, big toe, short fingers and large tongue [8]. DS patients may have an increased dosage or copy number that can lead to an increase in gene expression in Hsa 21 [8]. Specific genes such as Hsa21 or subsets of genes are able to control specific DS phenotypes [9]. In addition, phenotypic analyzes were performed on individuals with partial trisomy for Hsa21. It has been determined that a 3.8–6.5 Mb region called "Down syndrome critical regions" (DSCR) is responsible for most of the Down syndrome phenotypes at 21q21.22 [9]. With the sequencing of Hsa 21, more information was learned about DS-associated genotype–phenotype correlations and characterization of DSCR regions [3]. It has been suggested that the dual- specificity tyrosine phosphorylation-regulated kinase (DYRK1A), the regulator of calcineurin 1 (RCAN1) and Down syndrome cell adhesion molecule (DSCAM), play a critical role in brain development and the occurrence of heart defects in DS patients [10]. In particular, DSCAM plays a very important role in neuron differentiation, axon guidance and neural networks formation. Disruption of these processes contributes to the DS neurocognitive anomalies. All studies have shown that there is not a single critical gene region sufficient to cause DS phenotypes, and there must be a large number of critical regions or critical genes contributing to a DS-associated phenotype or phenotypes.

3. Various pheotypes associated to Down syndrome

The various clinical phenotypes associated with DS are Alzheimer's disease, heart defects, leukemia, hypertension and gastrointestinal problems (**Figure 2**).

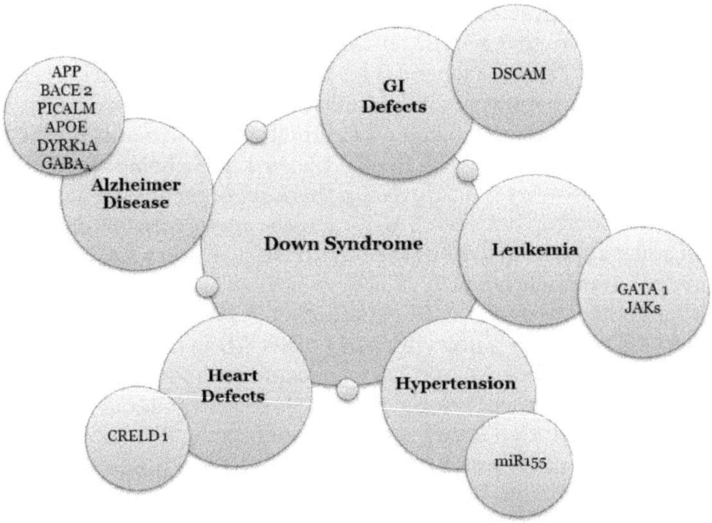

Figure 2.
Various phenotypes associated with Downs's syndrome with its responsible genes (GI: Gastrointestinal).

The pathogenesis mechanism of these phenotypes associated with DS should be studied together with their causative agents to better understand the disease.

3.1 Alzheimer disease

It has been determined that the risk of early onset Alzheimer Disease (AD) is high in DS patients. After the age of 50, the risk of developing dementia increases up to 70% in patients with DS [11]. In the past decade, substantial progress has been made in the search for genetic risk factors for dementia in people with DS, and in understanding the neuropathological similarities and differences between AD with DS and without DS. For people with DS over the age of 40, dementia development has a similar progression to that of AD [12–14]. However, if dementia occurs in younger individuals (30–40 years of age), it manifests itself as personality and behavior changes such as increasing impulsivity and onset of apathy [10]. The most conspicuous parallel between AD and AD in DS are characteristic neuropathologies such as amyloid-β accumulation [15]. Results from post-mortem neurochemistry studies have showed a significant loss of choline acetyltransferase and noradrenaline in people with DS, which is similar to the changes seen in Alzheimer's disease [16]. Results obtained from studies, the cholinergic dysregulation in DS is controlled by the DYRK1A gene [17]. DYRK1A is a serine–threonine protein kinase. DYRK1A is involved in tau phosphorylation, and it's up-regulation may contribute to early onset formation of neurofibrillary tangles. In addition, the results obtained from microarray studies, pointed out that there is an up-regulation of the α2 subunit and down-regulation of the α3 and α5 subunits of $GABA_A$ receptor [18].

There are several genes known to cause early onset AD. The most important of these genes are APP (amyloid precursor protein), BACE2 (beta secretase 2), PICALM (Phosphatidylinositol binding clathrin assembly protein) and APOE (Apolipoprotein E) [19, 20]. APP is an integral membrane protein concentrated in the synapse of neurons. It is thought that the trisomy of this protein may contribute significantly to the increased frequency of dementia in individuals with DS. It has been shown that trisomic of APP along with Hsa 21 in non-DS individuals is associated with early onset AD. In a preliminary study, a tetranucleotide repeat, ATTT, in intron 7 of the amyloid precursor protein, was associated with the onset of AD in DS [20]. It is also known that BACE2, encoding the enzyme beta secretase 2, plays a role in AD. Like APP, the BACE 2 gene is located on chromosome 21. The results of the studies are that the haplotypes in BACE2 are associated with AD [21]. A genome wide study, an important relationship was found between variants in BACE2 and age of onset of dementia in DS, with the rs2252576-T allele being associated with an earlier onset by 2–4 years [22]. However, there are other studies that reported no significant relationship between BACE2 and the age of onset of dementia [23]. There is still some uncertainty about the relationship between BACE2 variants and the development of dementia in DS.

In addition to the APP and BACE2 genes, other genes such as PICALM and APOE were found to be associated with early onset AD in DS [24]. PICALM, the other candidate risk gene for AD and DS were examined. PICALM is present in enlarged endosomes in early developing AD [25]. In a DS genome wide study, a relationship has been verified between the variation in the PICALM region of chromosome 11 and the age of onset of AD [26]. Three SNPS in this study, rs2888903, rs7941541 and rs10751134 has been associated with an earlier age of onset. The ε4 allele of the APOE gene, located on chromosome 19, is the most important genetic risk factor for late-onset Alzheimer's disease [27]. The APOE ε4 allele, known to be associated with increased amyloid burden and cholinergic dysfunction, is probably the most studied genetic risk factor. In individuals with DS, the presence of the APOE ε4 allele has been shown to increase the risk of Alzheimer's disease [28, 29]. Also, Aβ accumulation DS individuals carrying the APOE ε4 allele are increased [30].

3.2 Heart defects

The frequency of heart defects in newborns with DS is up to 50% [31]. The defect called atrioventricular cushion defect is the most common heart defect affecting 40% of DS patients. Ventricular septal defect (VSD) also affects 35% of patients [31]. In atrioventricular septal defect (AVSD), there is a common atrioventricular junction in contrast to normal heart. Other defects include muscular and membranous atrioventricular septum defects and an oval shape of the common atrioventricular junction. Pulmonary arterial hypertension occurs in 1.2 to 5.2% of people with DS [32]. Early repair of heart defects minimizes the risks of heart failure and irreversible pulmonary vascular disease [33]. Observation of specific anatomical patterns of heart defects that can be seen in DS showed that a locus on chromosome 21 plays a role in the development of cardiac malformations [34, 35]. Although up-regulation of genes mapped on chromosome 21 is thought to be related to heart defects, the molecular basis that regulating existence and anatomy of heart defects are still unclear [34]. It has been suggested that type VI collagen (COL6A1, COL6A2) is involved in the pathogenesis of AVSD in Down syndrome, in a similar way to other genes mapping on chromosome [36].

Apart from chromosome 21, other genes localized on different chromosomes have also been studied as the cause of heart defects in DS. Among these genes, the CRELD1 gene has been evaluated as increasing susceptibility to AVSD [31]. Mutations in the CRELD1 (Cysteine-rich EGF-like domain1) gene has been found to contribute to the development of AVSD in DS [37]. CRELD1 gene is located on chromosome 3p25 and contains 11 exons spanning approximately 12 kb [38]. This gene encodes a cell surface protein that functions as a cell adhesion molecule and is expressed during cardiac cushion development. There are studies suggesting that the CRELD1 gene probably plays a major role in the causation of the AVSD phenotype in DS individuals [39, 40]. Two heterozygous missense mutations (p.R329C and p.E414K) were identified with two subjects in DS and AVSD [31]. They also included 39 DS with complete AVSD and found the same mutations. No such mutation was detected in DS individuals without heart defects [37]. The R329C mutation reported in a person with sporadic partial AVSD and has also been detected in an individual with DS with AVSD. Although the mutation is the same in DS patients AVSD heart defect has created a more serious condition. Therefore, it has been suggested that the CRELD 1 mutation contributes to the pathogenesis of AVSD heart defects occurring in DS individuals.

3.3 Hypertension

Individuals with DS may have an increased risk of developing pulmonary hypertension (PH), in part due to congenital heart defects. Other factors such as upper airway obstruction, lung hypoplasia with DS, gastroesophageal reflux, abnormal pulmonary vascular function may play a role in increasing the risk of PH in DS. Findings from a study with DS in Mexico City (high altitude) showed that % 40 had congenital heart disease and 80% had PH [41, 42]. On the other hand, a reduced incidence of hypertension has been reported in individuals with DS [43, 44].

Some of the Hsa21-encoded miRs have been shown to be overexpressed in cells and tissues of DS patients. The direct cause of the overexpression of miRs in DS appears to be the extra copy of HSA21, whose miRs are at their normal chromosomal location [45]. It has been reported that trisomy of Hsa21 microRNA hsa-miR-155 causes this low incidence [45]. An allele of the type-1 angiotensin II receptor (AGTR1) gene is the specific target of HsamiR-155. In this study of twins (one twin was unaffected, and the other had a trisomy 21) to evaluate the expression of MiR-155 in trisomy 21, both twins are homozygous for the 1166A AGTR1 allele and therefore AGTR1 Reported to be the target of miR-155 [46]. This receptor has a vasopressor effect and regulates aldosterone secretion. It is an important factor controlling blood pressure and volume in the cardiovascular system. In this way, it is suggested that it contributes to the decrease of the risk of hypertension by reducing the expression of AGTR1. More studies are needed to validate these thoughts and to determine whether other genes could also protect DS people against hypertension.

3.4 Leukemia

Hematological abnormalities are common in patients with DS. Patients with DS have a wide risk of malignancy including leukemia. The first leukemia report in a DS patient was in 1930 [47]. It has been reported that leukemia may develop in DS individuals with subsequent systemic studies. Studies have shown that DS patients have an approximately 10–20 times higher risk of leukemia, with a 2% risk by age 5 and 2.7% at age 30 [48]. DS individuals account for about 2% of all childhood acute lymphoblastic leukemia (ALL) and about 10% of acute myeloid leukemia (AML).

Somatic mutations such as GATA 1 gene play a role in the development of acute megakaryoblastic leukemia (AMKL) in DS patients [49]. GATA 1 is a transcription factor localized on the X chromosome, which plays a role in erythroid and megakaryocytic differentiation. Mutations in GATA 1 cause a shorter GATA 1 protein to be expressed and consequently uncontrolled proliferation of immature megakaryocytes [49, 50]. Transient abnormal myelopoiesis, a form of myeloid preleukemia that occurs in about 10% of newborns with DS, is also caused by mutations in GATA1 [4]. A mutation in GATA1 in individuals with DS has been reported to cause transient myeloproliferative disorder (TMD) [51]. They thought it was likely that trisomy 21 and GATA1 causing hyperplasia of the fetal liver in some DS individuals to induce perinatal TMD.

Another mutation that has been suggested to play a role in ALL cases occurring in DS is in the Janus Kinase 2 (JAK 2) gene and is present in approximately 30% of ALL cases in DS [52]. Mutations in the JAK–STAT pathway are at high risk for the development of ALL in individuals with DS [53]. JAK2 is a non-receptor tyrosine kinase and a member of the Janus kinase family. It has been implicated in signaling by members of some receptor families (e.g. interferon receptors and interleukin receptors) [54]. Mutations in JAK2 have been associated with polycythemia vera, essential thrombocythemia, myelofibrosis, and other myeloproliferative disorders. Also, it has been reported that the JAK1, JAK2 and JAK3 genes are mutated in AMKL patients with DS [55–57].

3.5 Gastrointestinal defects

Individuals with DS consist about 12% of Hirschprung disease (HD) cases. HD is an intestinal obstruction caused by the absence of normal myenteric ganglion cells in part of the colon [58]. In this gastrointestinal (GI) defect, peristaltic waves do not pass through the aganglionic segment and cause obstruction as there is no normal defecation. Other GI defects that can be seen in individuals with DS are duodenal stenosis (DST) and imperforate anus (IA). They are seen 260 and 33 times more respectively in DS [59]. In newborns with duodenal blockage or DST, bilious vomiting occurs in the early neonatal period. If left untreated, there is a risk of death due to severe dehydration and electrolyte imbalance. IA is a birth defect that causes rectal malformation and is associated with the increase of some other specific anomalies such as tracheoesophageal fistula and esophageal atresia.

It has been suggested that changes in genes unrelated to Hsa21 play a role in these diseases. DSCAM has long been viewed as a candidate gene explaining the increased prevalence of this GI defect in HD patients with DS. DSCAM is Down syndrome cell adhesion molecule and plays a crucial role in the development of DS. It is a trans-membrane protein and a member of the immunoglobulin (Ig) superfamily of cell adhesion molecules. It is expressed in the developing nervous system with the highest level of expression occurring in the fetal brain. When over-expressed in the developing fetal central nervous system, it leads to Down syndrome. DSCAM gene is expressed in neural crest that gives rise to enteric nervous system. The overlapping critical region is defined for both DST and IA [58]. Alterations in the DSCAM gene have been shown to play a role in HD development. In connection with HD, two SNPs, rs2837770 and rs8134673, spanning a 19 kb exon-free region of the DSCAM gene was identified [60].

4. Conclusions

DS, the most common chromosomal abnormality among newborns, is associated with a number of congenital malformations, primarily mental retardation caused by the trisomy of chromosome 21. In addition to its own characteristics, DS can be accompanied by different phenotypes. Different theories such as "gene dosage" have been considered to understand the interactions between phenotype and genotype. The DS phenotype is mainly due to the dosage imbalance of genes located on human chromosome 21 (Hsa 21). The most common cause of DS is presence extra copy chromosome 21. A critical region in 21q22 is thought to be responsible for various DS phenotypes such as craniofacial abnormalities, congenital heart defects, clinodactyly and mental retardation. The health problems and life period of DS people are quite complex and are associated with many different medical, psychological and social problems from infancy to adulthood. In this chapter, it is to reveal the common genes involved in DS related phenotypes such as APP, BACE2, PICALM, APOE, GATA 1, JAK 2.

The association of DS with various clinical phenotypes requires continuous following of these patients with a multidisciplinary approach. For example, there are numerous epidemiological and molecular studies linking the pathological changes observed in the brains of individuals with Down syndrome and the neurodegeneration seen in Alzheimer's disease. Knowing the genes and pathology associated with such changes is very important for a good clinical follow-up of DS patients. Due to the insufficient knowledge of the molecular pathogenesis of DS, an effective therapeutic intervention is unlikely to be found yet. The situation is further complicated by the complex phenotypes accompanying DS. It may be a good option to use pharmacological approaches to key target molecules that are crucial for dysregulated metabolic pathways or phenotypic characteristics. In conclusion, elucidating the phenotypic consequences of gene dose imbalance in DS and knowing the genes that cause accompanying phenotypes may provide new opportunities for therapeutic interventions.

Author details

Fatma Söylemez
Department of Food Processing, Vocational School of Technical Sciences, Mersin University, Mersin, Turkey

*Address all correspondence to: soylemez_fatma@yahoo.com

References

[1] Sherman SL, Allen EG, Bean LH, Freeman SB. Epidemiology of Down sydrome. Mental Retardation and Developmental Disabilities Research Reviews, 13: 221-227, 2007.

[2] Soylemez F. Double Aneuploidy in Down Syndrome. Health Problems in Down Syndrome. InTechOpen, Chapter 6, 101-123, 2015.

[3] Antonarakis SE, Lyle R, Dermitzakis ET, Reymond A, Deutsch S. Chromosome 21 and Down syndrome: from genomics to pathophysiology. Nat Rev Genetics, 5: 725-738, 2004.

[4] Bull MJ. Down Syndrome. The New England Journal of Medicine, 382: 2344-2352, 2020.

[5] Asim A, Kumar A, Muthuswamy S, Jain S, Agarwal S. Down syndrome: an insight of the disease. Journal of Biomedical Science, 22: 41-50, 2015.

[6] Mégarbané A, Ravel A, Mircher C, Sturtz F, Grattau Y, Rethoré MO, Delabar JM, Mobley WC. The 50th anniversary of the discovery of trisomy 21: the past, present, and future of research and treatment of Down syndrome. Genet Med, 11: 611-616, 2009.

[7] Prandini P, Deutsch S, Lyle R, Gagnebin M, Delucinge Vivier C, Delorenzi M, Gehrig C, Descombes P, Sherman S, Bricarelli FD, Baldo C, Novelli A, Dallapiccola B, Antonarakis SE. Natural gene-expression variation in Down syndrome modulates the outcome of gene-dosage imbalance. Am J Hum Genet, 81: 252-263, 2007.

[8] Patterson D. Genetic mechanisms involved in the phenotype of Down syndrome. Ment Retard Dev Disabil Res Rev, 3: 199-206, 2007.

[9] Pritchard MA, Kola I. The "gene dosage effect" hypothesis versus the "amplified developmental instability" hypothesis in Down syndrome. J Neural Transm Suppl, 57: 293-303, 1999.

[10] Holland AJ, Hon J, Huppert FA, Stevens F. Incidence and course of dementia in people with Down's syndrome: findings from a population based study. J Intellect Disabil Res, 44: 138-146, 2000.

[11] Janicki MP, Dalton AJ. Prevalence of dementia and impact on intellectual disability services. Ment Retard, 38: 276-288, 2000.

[12] Ballard C, Mobley W, Hardy J, Williams G, Corbett A. Dementia in Down's syndrome. Lancet Neurol, 15: 622-636, 2016.

[13] Holland AJ, Hon J, Huppert FA, Stevens F, Watson P. Population-based study of the prevalence and presentation of dementia in adults with Down's syndrome. Br J Psychiatry, 172: 493-498, 1998.

[14] Oliver C, Crayton L, Holland A, Hall S, Bradbury J. A four year prospective study of age-related cognitive change in adults with Down's syndrome. Psychol Med, 28: 1365-1377, 1998.

[15] Mann DM, Royston MC, Ravindra CR. Some morphometric observations on the brains of patients with Down's syndrome: their relationship to age and dementia. J Neurol Sci, 99: 153-164, 1990.

[16] Godridge H, Reynolds GP, Czudek C, Calcutt NA, Benton M. Alzheimer-like neurotransmitter deficits in adult Down's syndrome brain tissue. J Neurol Neurosurg Psychiatry, 50: 775-178, 1987.

[17] Hijazi M, Fillat C, Medina JM, Velasco A. Overexpression of DYRK1A inhibits choline acetyltransferase induction by oleic acid in cellular models of Down syndrome. Exp Neurol, 239: 229-234, 2013.

[18] Bhattacharyya A, McMillan E, Chen SI, Wallace K, Svendsen CN. A critical period in cortical interneuron neurogenesis in down syndrome revealed by human neural progenitor cells. Dev Neurosci, 31: 497-510, 2009.

[19] Myllykangas L, Wavrant–De Vrieze F, Polvikoski T, Notkola IL, Sulkava R, Niinisto L. Chromosome 21 BACE2 haplotype associates with Alzheimer's disease: a two-stage study. J Neurol Sci, 236 (1-2): 17-24, 2005.

[20] Jones EL, Ballard CG, Prasher VP, Arno M, Tyrer S, Moore B, Hanney ML. An Intron 7 polymorphism in APP affects the age of Dimentia in Down Syndrome. Int J Alzheimers Dis, 2011: 1-5, 2010.

[21] Myllykangas L, Wavrant-De Vrieze F, Polvikoski T, Notkola IL, Sulkava R, Niinisto L. Chromosome 21 BACE2 haplotype associates with Alzheimer's disease: a two-stage study. J Neurol Sci, 236 (1-2): 17-24, 2005.

[22] Mok KY, Jones EL, Hanney M, Harold D, Sims R, Williams J, Ballard C, Hardy J. Polymorphisms in BACE2 may affect the age of onset Alzheimer's dementia in Down syndrome. Neurobiol Aging, 35: 1513-1518, 2014.

[23] Yu Y, Jia J. Lack of association between the polymorphisms of beta-site APP-cleaving enzyme 2 (BACE2) 5′-flanking region and sporadic Alzheimer's disease. Brain Res, 1257: 10-15, 2009.

[24] Jones EL, Mok K, Hanney M, Harold D, Sims R, Williams J. Evidence that PICALM affects age at onset of Alzheimer's dementia in Down syndrome. Neurobiol Aging, 34 (10): 244, 2013.

[25] Cataldo AM, Peterhoff CM, Troncoso JC, Gomez-Isla T, Hyman BT, Nixon RA. Endocytic pathway abnormalities precede amyloid beta deposition in sporadic Alzheimer's disease and Down syndrome: differential effects of APOE genotype and presenilin mutations. Am J Pathol, 157: 277-286, 2000.

[26] Jones EL, Mok K, Hanney M, Harold D, Sims R, Williams J, Ballard C. Evidence that PICALM affects age at onset of Alzheimer's dementia in Down syndrome. Neurobiol Aging, 34: 2441, 1-5, 2013.

[27] Roses AD, Saunders AM, Corder EH, Pericak-Vance MA, Han SH, Einstein G, Hulette C, Schmechel DE, Holsti M, Huang D. Influence of the susceptibility genes apolipoprotein E-epsilon 4 and apolipoprotein E-epsilon 2 on the rate of disease expressivity of late-onset Alzheimer's disease. Arzneimittel-Forschung, 45: 413-417, 1995.

[28] Cedazo-Minguez A. Apolipoprotein E and Alzheimer's disease: molecular mechanisms and therapeutic opportunities. J Cell Mol Med, 11: 1227-1238, 2007.

[29] Deb S, Braganza J, Norton N, Williams H, Kehoe PG, Williams J, Owen MJ. APOE epsilon 4 influences the manifestation of Alzheimer's disease in adults with Down's syndrome. Br J Psychiatry, 176: 468-472, 2000.

[30] Hyman BT, West HL, Rebeck GW, Buldyrev SV, Mantegna RN, Ukleja M, Havlin S, Stanley HE. Quantitative analysis of senile plaques in Alzheimer disease: observation of log-normal size distribution and molecular epidemiology of differences associated with apolipoprotein E genotype and

trisomy 21 (Down syndrome). Proc Natl Acad Sci USA, 92: 3586-3590, 1995.

[31] Maslen CL, Babcock D, Robinson SW, Bean LJ, Dooley KJ, Willour VL, Sherman SL. CRELD1 mutations contribute to the occurrence of cardiac atrioventricular septal defects in Down syndrome. Am J Med Genet, 140: 2501-2505, 2006.

[32] Weijerman ME, van Furth AM, van der Mooren MD, van Weissenbruch MM, Rammeloo L, Broers CJM, Gemke RJB. Prevalence of congenital heart defects and persistent pulmonary hypertension of the neonate with Down syndrome. Eur J Pediatr, 169: 1195-1199, 2010.

[33] Martin T, Smith A, Breatnach CR, Kent E, Shanahan I, Boyle M, Levy PT, Franklin O, El-Khuffash A. Infants born with Down syndrome: burden of disease in the early neonatal period. J Pediatr, 193: 21-26, 2018.

[34] Versaccia P, Di Carloa D, Digiliob MC, Marino B. Cardiovascular disease in Down syndrome. Current Opinion in Pediatrics, 30 (5), 616-622, 2018.

[35] Korenberg JR, Bradley C, Disteche CM. Down syndrome: molecular mapping of the congenital heart disease and duodenal stenosis. Am J Hum Genet, 50: 294-302, 1992.

[36] Gittenberger-de Groot AC, Bartram U, Oosthoek PW, Bartelings MM, Hogers B, Poelmann RE, Jongewaard IN, Klewer SE. Collagen type VI expression during cardiac development and in human fetuses with trisomy 21. Anat Rec A Discov Mol Cell Evol Biol, 275: 1109-1116, 2003.

[37] Rup PA, Fouad GT, Egelston CA, Reifsteck CA, Oslon SB, Knosp WM, Glanville RW, Thornburg KL, Robinson SW, Maslen CL. Identification, genomic organization and mRNA expression of CRELD1, the founding member of a unique family of matricellular proteins. Gene, 293: 47-57, 2002.

[38] Sheffield VC, Pierpont ME, Nishimura D, Beek JS, Burns TL, Berg MA, Stone EM, Patil SR, Lauer RM. Identification of a complex congenital heart defect susceptibility locus by using DNA pooling and shared segment analysis. Hum Mol Genet, 6: 117-121, 1997.

[39] Asim A, Agarwal S, Panigrahi I, Sarangi AN, Muthuswamy S, Kapoor A. CRELD1 gene variants and atrioventricular septal defects in Down syndrome. Gene, 641: 180-185, 2018.

[40] Ghosh P, Bhaumik P, Ghosh S, Ozbek U, Feingold E, Maslen C, Sarkar B, Pramanik V, Biswas P, Bandyopadhyay B, Kumar Dey S. Polymorphic haplotypes of CRELD1 differentially predispose Down syndrome and euploids individuals to atrioventricular septal defect. Am J Med Genet A, 158A (11): 2843-2848, 2012.

[41] Beghetti M, Rudzinski A, Zhang M. Efficacy and safety of oral sildenafil in children with Down syndrome and pulmonary hypertension. BMC Cardiovascular Disorders, 17: 177-186, 2017.

[42] Espinola-Zavaleta N, Soto ME, Romero-Gonzalez A, Gomez-Puente, Gómez-Puente LDC, Munoz-Castellanos L, Gopal AS, Keirns C, Lupi-Herrera E. Prevalence of congenital heart disease and pulmonary hypertension in Down's syndrome: an Echocardiographic study. J Cardiovasc Ultrasound, 23: 72-77, 2015.

[43] Draheim CC, McCubbin JA, Williams DP. Differences in cardiovascular disease risk between nondiabetic adults with mental retardation with and without Down

syndrome. Am J Ment Retard, 107: 201-211, 2002.

[44] Sethupathy P, Borel C, Gagnebin M, Grant GR, Deutsch S, Elton TS, Hatzigeorgiou AG, Antonarakis SE. Human microRNA-155 on chromosome 21 differentially interacts with its polymorphic target in the AGTR1 3′ untranslated region: a mechanism for functional single-nucleotide polymorphisms related to phenotypes. Am J Hum Genet, 81: 405-413, 2007.

[45] Farroni C, Marasco E, Marcellini V, Giorda E, Valentini D, Petrini S, D'Oria V, Pezzullo M, Cascioli S, Scarsella M, Ugazio AG, De Vincentiis GC, Grimsholm O, Carsetti R. Dysregulated miR-155 and miR-125b Are Related to Impaired B-cell Responses in Down Syndrome. Front Immunol, 9: 2683-2695, 2018.

[46] Sethupathy P, Borel C, Gagnebin M, Grant GR, Deutsch S, Elton TS, Hatzigeorgiou AG, Antonarakis SE. Human microRNA-155 on Chromosome 21 Differentially Interacts with Its Polymorphic Target in the AGTR1 3 Untranslated Region: A Mechanism for Functional Single-Nucleotide Polymorphisms Related to Phenotypes. The American Journal of Human Genetics, 81 (2): 405-413, 2007.

[47] Brewster HF, Cannon HE. Acute lymphatic leukemia: Report of a case in eleventh month mongolina idiot. New Orleans Med Surg J, 82: 872-873, 1930.

[48] Hasle H, Clemmensen IH, Mikkelsen M. Risks of leukaemia and solid tumors in individuals with Down's syndrome. Lancet, 355: 165-169, 2000.

[49] Wechsler J, Greene M, McDevitt MA, Anastasi J, Karp JE, Le Beau MM, Crispino JD. Acquired mutations in GATA1 in the megakaryoblastic leukemia of Down syndrome. Nat Genet, 32 (1): 148-152, 2002.

[50] Shivdasani RA, Fujiwara Y, McDevitt MA, Orkin SH. A lineage-selective knockout establishes the critical role of transcription factor GATA-1 in megakaryocyte growth and platelet development. EMBO J, 16 (13): 3965-3973, 1997.

[51] Marshall GM, Carter DR, Cheung BB, Liu T, Mateos MK, Meyerowitz JG, Weiss WA. The prenatal origins of cancer. Nat Rev Cancer, 14 (4): 277-289, 2014.

[52] Kearney L, Gonzalez De Castro D, Yeung J, Procter J, Horsley SW, Eguchi-Ishimae M, Bateman CM, Anderson K, Chaplin T, Young BD, Harrison CJ, Kempski H, So CWE, Ford AM, Greaves M. Specific JAK2 mutation (JAK2R683) andmultiple gene deletions in Down syndrome acute lymphoblastic leukemia. Blood, 113 (3): 646-648, 2009.

[53] Mateos MK, Barbaric D, Byatt SA, Sutton R, Marshall GM. Down syndrome and leukemia: insights into leukemogenesis and translational targets. Transl Pediatr, 4 (2): 76-92, 2015.

[54] Brooks AJ, Dai W, O'Mara ML, Abankwa D, Chhabra Y, Pelekanos RA, Gardon O, Tunny KA, Blucher KM, Morton CJ, Parker MW, Sierecki E, Gambin Y, Gomez GA, Alexandrov K, Wilson IA, Doxastakis M, Mark AE, Waters MJ. Mechanism of activation of protein kinase JAK2 by the growth hormone receptor. Science, 344 (6185): 703-717, 2014.

[55] Yoshida K, Toki T, Okuno Y, Kanezaki R, Shiraishi Y, Sato-Otsubo A, Sanada M, Park M, Terui K, Suzuki H, Kon A, Nagata Y, Sato Y, Wang R, Shiba N, Chiba K, Tanaka H, Hama A, Muramatsu H, Hasegawa D, Nakamura K, Kanegane H,

Tsukamoto K, Adachi S, Kawakami K, Kato K, Nishimura R, Izraeli S, Hayashi Y, Miyano S, Kojima S, Ito E, Ogawa S. The landscape of somatic mutations in Down syndrome–related myeloid disorders. Nature Genetics, 45 (11): 1293-1299, 2013.

[56] Blink M, Buitenkamp TD, van den Heuvel-Eibrink MM, Danen-van Oorschot AA, de Haas V, Reinhardt D, Klusmann JH, Zimmermann M, Devidas M, Carroll AJ, Basso G, Pession A, Hasle H, Pieters R, Rabin KR, Izraeli S, Zwaan CM. Frequency and prognostic implications of JAK 1-3 aberrations in Down syndrome acute lymphoblastic and myeloid leukemia. Leukemia, 25: 1365-1368, 2011.

[57] Hama A, Muramatsu H, Makishima H, Sugimoto Y, Szpurka H, Jasek M, O'Keefe C, Takahashi Y, Sakaguchi H, Doisaki S, Shimada A, Watanabe N, Kato K, Kiyoi H, Naoe T, Kojima S, Maciejewski JP. Molecular lesions in childhood and adult acute megakaryoblastic leukaemia. Br. J. Haematol, 156: 316-325, 2012.

[58] Amiel J, Sproat-Emison E, Garcia-Barcelo M, Lantieri F, Burzynski G, Borrego S, Pelet A, Arnold S, Miao X, Griseri P, Brooks AS, Antinolo G, de Pontual L, Clement-Ziza M, Munnich A, Kashuk C, West K, Wong KY, Lyonnet S, Chakravarti A, Tam PKH, Ceccherini I, Hofstra RMW, Fernandez R. Hirschsprung disease, associated syndromes and genetics: a review. J Med Genet, 45: 1-14, 2008.

[59] Berrocal T, Lamas M, Gutiérrez J. Congenital Anomalies of the Small Intestine, Colon, and Rectum. Radiographics Radiol Bras, 19: 1219-1236, 1999.

[60] Jannot AS, Pelet A, Henrion-Caude A, Chaoui A, Morel M, Arnold S, Sanlaville D, Ceccherini I, Borrego S, Hofstra RMW, Munnich A, Bondurand N, Chakravarti A, Clerget-Darpoux F, Amiel J, Lyonne S. Chromosome 21 Scan in Down Syndrome Reveals DSCAM as a Predisposing Locus in Hirschsprung Disease. PLoS One, 8 (5): 1-8, 2013.

Section 4

Haematological Malignancies and Congenital Heart Disease in Down Syndrome

Chapter 7

Chromosome Abnormalities in Hematological Malignancies and Its Clinical Significance

Hariharan Sreedharan

Abstract

The latest version of the World Health Organization guidelines focuses mainly on the genetic and cytogenetic features of hematologic neoplasms as predictors of diagnostic, treatment decision, prognostic outcome, and for treatment monitoring in hematological malignancies. There are different techniques to identify these abnormalities. Live cells are needed for chromosome preparation. The Hematological malignancies include myeloid and lymphoid neoplasms. The myeloid neoplasms include Myelodysplastic syndromes, myeloproliferative neoplasms, and acute myeloid leukemias. The Lymphoid neoplasms include acute and chronic lymphocytic leukemias, plasma cell neoplasms, myeloma, hodgkin, and non-hodgkin lymphomas. The first chromosomal abnormality discovered in connection with cancer is the Philadelphia chromosome, which is an abnormal chromosome 22, formed due to the translocation between chromosomes 9 and 22. The presence of this abnormal chromosome confirms the diagnosis of "CML". After that, hundreds of chromosomal abnormalities have been identified in hematological malignancies in different parts of the world. In AML, specific abnormalities were identified as having a good prognosis, intermediate prognosis, and poor prognosis. In other hematological malignancies also there some specific chromosome abnormalities are associated with prognostication. Now a day's clinicians depend mainly on genetic abnormalities for the proper treatment management of hematological malignancies, so the study of chromosomal abnormalities is essential.

Keywords: hematological malignancies, chromosomes, abnormalities, cytogenetics, karyotype, leukemia, lymphoma

1. Introduction

In hematological malignancies, the study of chromosomal abnormalities is essential for the proper diagnosis, prognosis prediction, treatment decision, and treatment monitoring. The important technique used for the study of chromosomal abnormalities are the conventional cytogenetics, the advanced techniques like Fluorescent In situ Hybridization (FISH), Spectral Karyotyping (SKY)/ Multiplex Karyotyping/MFISH, and, to some extent, array comparative genomic hybridization (array CGH), have enhanced the knowledge of chromosome abnormalities in hematologic neoplasms [1]. The cytogenetic study requires the presence of live cells or at least intact nuclei. Human cancer cells divide spontaneously and without culturing, chromosomes could be prepared from the sample [2]. These

IntechOpen

techniques have contributed immensely to the discovery of significant cryptic rearrangements in various tissue preparations of leukemia and other cancers. The advanced techniques in cytogenetics FISH, SKY, and CGH are seen as a potential competitor to conventional cytogenetics, due to their higher resolution. Still conventional cytogenetic analysis remains as the best method for the diagnosis of most hematologic neoplasms since it has the advantage of an overall examination of all chromosomes at a glance. Conventional cytogenetics help to identify distinct clonal populations, which are not possible by FISH and practically impossible by array CGH [3, 4].

2. Myeloid neoplasms

Myelodysplastic syndromes (MDS), Myeloproliferative neoplasms (MPN), MDS/MPN, and acute myeloid leukemias are included in this group. The classification of myeloid neoplasms has recently been modified considering the genetic and cytogenetic abnormalities [5].

2.1 Myelodysplastic syndromes (MDS)

MDS is a heterogeneous group of hematopoietic neoplasms with an increased risk of transformation into acute myeloid leukemia (AML) via a multistep process [6]. Chromosomal studies are essential for both diagnostic and prognostic information. In about 50% of patients chromosome abnormalities could be observed. The severity of the disease is associated with the frequency of chromosomal abnormalities [7, 8]. About 25% of patients with low-grade MDS, such as refractory anemia and refractory anemia with ring sideroblasts, have an abnormal karyotype, compared with 50–70% of patients with refractory anemia with excess blasts (RAEB-1 and RAEB-2). The karyotypes observed in MDS are variable as they present with single or complex chromosome rearrangements [9, 10]. The most frequent chromosome abnormalities are complete or partial loss of chromosomes 5 and/or 7, deletions on the long arm of chromosome 20, and gain of chromosome 8 [11]. In general, aggressive neoplasms are characterized by more complex karyotypes than those seen in low-grade MDS. Furthermore, as a general rule, dosage aberrations appear to be more represented in primary MDS, whereas balanced translocations are encountered more frequently in secondary MDS. Complex karyotypes with loss/deletion of chromosomes 5 and/or 7 together with deletions of 6p, 12p, and/or 16q are typical in therapy-related MDS, whereas balanced translocations involving 11q23 and 21q22.3 are associated with preceding therapy with DNA topoisomerase II inhibitors [12]. According to the presence of chromosome abnormalities, MDS is classified into different risk groups. 12p-, 9q-, t(15q), 15q-, +21, 5q-, 20q-, -X, -Y, t(19), t(7q), -21 and normal Karyotype are considered as good prognosis. Patients with abnormalities +8,11q-, +18 are included in the Intermediate I group. The presence of abnormalities like t(11q23), any 3q abnormality, +19, 7q-, complex abnormalities (less than 3 abnormalities) are included in the Intermediate II group. Complex abnormalities (more than 3 abnormalities), 3q21.3q26.2, t(5q), 7q/monosomy 7 are considered as poor prognosis [13]. The significance of trisomy 15 with or without the loss of the Y chromosome is not fully understood. Apparently balanced translocations have been reported in MDS, involved with chromosomes 1, 2, 3, 5, 6, 7, 13, 15, 17, 18, 19, and 20 appear to be more frequent, but they appear to be less common than the unbalanced rearrangements [14].

2.2 Myeloproliferative neoplasms (MPNs)

Myeloproliferative neoplasms are hematopoietic stem cell disorders characterized by the proliferation of one or more myeloid cellular elements in the marrow and mostly affect adult individuals. Chronic myelogenous leukemia (CML), polycythemia vera (PV), primary myelofibrosis (PMF), essential thrombocythemia (ET), chronic eosinophilic leukemia (CEL), systemic mastocytosis, chronic neutrophilic leukemia (CNL), and the unclassifiable MPNs [5].

2.3 Chronic myelogenous leukemia

Chronic myelogenous leukemia (CML) is a hematopoietic stem cell disease, most frequently seen in adults. It is characterized by a biphasic or triphasic clinical course in which a benign chronic phase is followed by transformation into an accelerated and blastic phase [15, 16]. The hallmark of CML is the presence of the "Philadelphia chromosome" (Ph), which is the first chromosome abnormality identified to have been associated with a specific malignant neoplasm. The Ph chromosome was first described in 1960 by Nowell and Hungerford and is named after the city in which it was discovered [17]. Because of a reciprocal translocation between chromosome 9 and 22; a major portion from the q arm of chromosome 22 is translocated to the q arm of chromosome 9 and a small portion from the q arm of 9 is translocate the q arm of 22, leads to a shortened chromosome 22, called the Philadelphia chromosome. The t (9;22) (q34;q11.2), leads to the formation of a chimeric transcript between the *ABL1* and *BCR* genes at 9q34 and 22q11.2, respectively [18]. This BCR-ABL fusion gene formed in chromosome 22 is responsible for CML. The main abnormality seen in the chronic phase of CML is t(9;22). Variant translocation due to the involvement of one or more additional chromosomes is observed in about 6% of cases, whereas in approximately 3% of cases the translocation cannot be identified by routine cytogenetics [19]. These variants and cryptic rearrangements generally have the same prognostic outcome of the standard t(9;22), but some are associated with a more aggressive course. Conventional cytogenetic analysis can sometimes reveal abnormalities in addition to the t(9;22). It is important to note, however, that an additional balanced rearrangement in all metaphase cells in chronic phase CML might be constitutional in origin. Additional abnormalities are associated with the accelerated phase or blast crisis, and are characterized by an increase in the number of blasts and worsening of clinical symptoms [20]. The most recurrent chromosome abnormalities (about 90% of cases) in these phases are an additional Ph chromosome, +8, i(17) (q10), and/or +19. Other abnormalities, such as −Y, −7, +21, +19,del(7q), 11q23 del, t(8;21)(q22;q22.3), t(15;17) (q24.1;q21.2), inv.(16)(p13.1q22.1), as well as 3q21.3, 3q26.2, 3 way Ph, 4 way Ph and 11q23 rearrangements have been reported but only in a small number of cases [21].

2.4 Polycythemia vera (PV)

PV is most commonly seen in men over the age of 50, but anyone can develop PV. These patients typically experience an increased number of white blood cells, an increased platelet count, and an enlarged spleen, especially over time, which in some patients leads to bleeding and thrombosis [22]. About 14–20% of patients with PV have karyotypic abnormalities at the time of initial diagnosis. However, the cytogenetic abnormalities in PV have not been well characterized and their prognosis impact is largely unknown. At the chromosome level, patients are *BCR-ABL* fusion-negative, other abnormalities detected are +1, +8, +9/+9p, and/or del (20q). Furthermore, a gain of 9p is usually the result of a derivative chromosome, the most common of which is a der (9; 18) (p10; q10). This gain is often the result of unbalanced translocations. When the disease progresses abnormalities like del (5q), del (7q), and/or del (17p) appear [23–25].

2.5 Primary myelofibrosis (PM)

Primary myelofibrosis, also known as idiopathic myelofibrosis and agnogenic myeloid metaplasia, is characterized by an increased number of megakaryocytes and immature granulocytes and associated anemia. Affected patients are generally in their 5th and 6th decade of life [26]. Chromosome abnormalities are observed in about 40–50% of cases at diagnosis. del(13q), del(20q), and gain of chromosome 8 are the commonly seen abnormalities, and additional abnormalities such as del (5q), del (7q), gain of 1q, and del (17p) are detected during disease progression [27].

2.6 Essential thrombocythemia (ET)

ET is most commonly seen in women over the age of 50, characterized by an increased number of platelets in the peripheral blood. Chromosome abnormalities could be seen in about 10% of cases. The commonly seen abnormalities are +8, +9, del(13q), and del(20q), less commonly gain of 1q, del(5q), and del(7q). As in other MPNs, karyotypic abnormalities are more frequent during disease progression to MDS or AML [28].

2.7 Systemic mastocytosis (SM)

Systemic mastocytosis, often termed systemic mast cell disease (SMCD), is characterized by infiltration of clonally derived mast cells in different tissues, including bone marrow, skin, the gastrointestinal (GI) tract, the liver, and the spleen [29]. Most Patients with systemic mastocytosis (SM) are characterized by symptoms such as hepatomegaly, osteoporosis, and ascites. This is a very complex disease, as it comprises several distinct entities and is also found in association with neoplasms such as MPN and leukemia [29]. Chromosome abnormalities reported are +8, +9, del(7q), del(11q), del(20q), t(8;21), inv.(16)/t(16;16) and rearrangements involving chromosome 4 [30].

2.8 Chronic neutrophilic leukemia (CNL)

CNL is a rare *BCR-ABL* negative myeloproliferative neoplasm (MPN) characterized by sustained, predominantly mature neutrophil proliferation, bone marrow granulocytic hyperplasia, and hepatosplenomegaly. As the name implies, it is characterized by an increase in the number of mature neutrophils [31]. Approximately 20% of cases have an abnormal karyotype. The abnormalities observed so far include +8, +9, del(11q), del(20q), +21, and less frequently del(12p) [32].

2.9 Chronic myelomonocytic leukemia (CMML)

CMML happens when monocytes in the bone marrow begin to grow out of control and is characterized by persistent monocytosis and a variable degree of dysplasia [33]. Although no specific abnormality has been associated with CMML, recurrent chromosome abnormalities, such as −7/del(7q), a gain of chromosome 8, and less commonly del(5q), 12p rearrangements, i(17)(q10) and t(5;12)(q33.1;p13.2) have been observed [34].

2.10 Juvenile myelomonocytic leukemia (JMML)

JMML is a rare MPN that predominantly affects young children under the age of four, characterized by an abnormal proliferation of myelocytes and monocytes in the bone marrow [35]. The most common abnormality is −7/del (7q) and less frequently del(5q). The final diagnosis is based on the exclusion of the translocation 9:22 [36, 37].

2.11 Acute myeloid leukemia (AML)

AML is characterized by an increase in the number of myeloid cells in the marrow and an arrest in their maturation, frequently resulting in hematopoietic insufficiency, with or without leukocytosis. At least 20% of blasts should be present in the marrow. The classification AML has been revised by the WHO by considering the various genetic and cytogenetic changes. Although AML more frequently affects adults in their 5th decade of life, it has been described in children and young adults also [38]. AML is associated with characteristic recurrent, acquired chromosomal abnormalities, and many are reciprocal translocations that generate a fusion gene, others involve partial or complete loss or gain of a chromosome. Cytogenetic findings are important for the diagnosis and classification of AML and some are associated with distinctive clinicopathologic features, have prognostic significance, and /or influence in the choice of therapy [39]. Recurrent Genetic Abnormalities seen in AML are t(8;21)(q22;q22.3), inv.(16) (p13.1q22.1) or (16;16)(p13.1;q22.1), t(15;17)(q24.1;q21.2), t(9;11)(p22;q23), t(6;9)(p23;q34.1), inv.(3)(q21.3q26.2) or t(3;3)(q21.3;q26.2), and t(1;22)(p13.3;q13.1). As per WHO classification, AML is classified into good, intermediate, and poor prognostic categories according to the presence of specific chromosomal abnormalities [40]. The abnormalities associated with favorable outcome in AML are t(8;21)(q22;q22.3), inv.(16)(p13.1q22.1) or t(16;16)(p13.1;q22.1), t(15;17) (q24.1;q21.2) Intermediate prognosis group include t(9;11)(p21.3;q23.3), adverse group are t(6;9)(p23.1;q34.1), t(v; 11q23.3), t(9;22) (q34.1;q11.2), inv.(3)q21.3;) or t(3;3), −5 or del(5q), −7, −17, abn(17p), complex karyotype and monosomy karyotype. The presence of additional abnormalities in patients with good prognostic features changes the overall disease prognosis. The most frequent additional abnormality in patients with t(8;21) is loss of a sex chromosome (the Y in males), followed by del(9q), del(7q), +8, and/or +21. Other additional chromosome abnormalities seen in patients with inv.(16) include +8, del(7q), and/or + 21and +22 [41, 42]. Acute Promyelocytic Leukemia (APML), is a subtype of AML with the recurrent abnormality t(15;17) (q24.1;q21.2). Originally considered one of the most aggressive leukemias, it is now a model for targeted therapy. Additional abnormalities frequently been observed in *APL*, are +8, del(9q), and del(7q) [43]. In about 5-10 % AML patients, MLL rearrangements at 11q23 could be seen. Among the identified 85 known *MLL* translocations, the majority are of with poor outcomes. Other frequent *MLL* translocation are t(11;19), t(6;11)(q27;q23), t(10;11)(q21.3;q23), inv.(3)(q21.3q26.2) or t(3;3) (q 21.3;q 26.2). The most common additional abnormalities that are seen in cases with rearrangements of 3q21.3 and 3q26.2 are −7 and, less frequently, del(5q) [44, 45].

2.12 Acute megakaryoblastic leukemia (AMKL)

AMKL is a clonal stem cell neoplasm that comprises between 4%and 15% of newly diagnosed pediatric AML patients [46]. This is commonly regarded as a subtype of AML, with the median age at presentation between 1 and 8 years. AMKL is extremely rare in adults, occurring in only 1% of AML cases. In pediatrics this disease is divided into two major subgroups: AMKL patients with Down Syndrome (DSAMKL) and AMKL patients without DS (non-DS AMKL). The incidence of developing DS- AMKL is 500 fold higher than in the general population [46]. The main abnormality seen is t (1; 22) which is diagnostic in this group and is considered as with intermediate prognosis. Chromosome abnormalities at diagnosis are observed in about 50% of adult patients and the most common rearrangements seen are in regions 3q21.3 and 3q26.2. Other abnormalities seen frequently are −5/del(5q), −7/del(7q), and +8 [46].

2.13 Myeloid sarcoma (MS)

Myeloid sarcoma or granulocytic sarcoma is a rare disease that can present as an extramedullary leukemic tumor, concurrently with or at relapse of AML. This is also known as chloroma, although in some rare cases it may present in non-leukemic patients also [47]. MS may be common in patients included in FAB class M2, WHO classification (2016) in a separate entity under 'AML and related neoplasms' and those with cytogenetic abnormalities t(8;21) or inv.(16). The common cytogenetic abnormalities observed in myeloid sarcoma are −7, +8, del(5q), del(20q), +4, +11, del(12p), del(16q), del(13q), del(9p), del(9q), del(6q), del(15q), del(4q), inv.(16)/t(16;16), MLL rearrangements, and t(8;21)(q22;q22.3). The prognosis is variable as it is influenced by several factors including but not limited to age, morphology, and cytogenetic abnormality [48–50].

3. Lymphoid neoplasms

Lymphoid neoplasms are derived from cells that normally develop into T Lymphocytes or B Lymphocytes (lymphocytes or plasma cells). This includes Acute and chronic lymphocytic leukemias, plasma cell neoplasms, myeloma, Hodgkin and Non-Hodgkin lymphomas. This group of hematologic neoplasms includes immature and mature neoplasms of B-cell, T-cell, and natural killer (NK) cell subtypes [51, 52]. This leukemia is more common in children than in adults. The majority of lymphoid neoplasms (both precursor and mature types) are characterized by recurrent chromosome abnormalities [53].

3.1 Acute lymphoid neoplasms

This neoplasm is defined as leukemia when it involves the bone marrow and peripheral blood and as lymphoma when it presents as a lesion without evidence of bone marrow and peripheral blood involvement. Approximately 85% of B-ALL patients are children [53–55]. Chromosome abnormalities are useful for prognostic stratification in acute neoplasms. Abnormalities like t(9;22)(q34;q11.2), 11q23 (MLL) rearrangements, t(1;19)(q23.3;p13.3), and hypodiploidy (≤45 chromosomes) in children are known to have an unfavorable prognosis, whereas t(12;21)(p13.2;q22.3) and hyperdiploidy (>50 chromosomes) are associated with a favorable prognostic outcome. t(9;22) (q34;q11.2) appears in approximately 2.5% of children and approximately 25% of adults with B-ALL [56, 57] . Chromosome abnormalities in addition to the t(9;22) are seen in more than 60% of patients, specifically +8 and one extra copy of the Ph chromosome. Other abnormalities seen in B-ALL are −7, +X, and del(9p). MLL translocations are also found BLL which include t(4;11) (q21.3;q23), t(11;19) (q23;p13.3), t(6;11)(q27;q230 and t(9;11)(p22;q23) [58–61]. MLL rearrangements are associated with an unfavorable prognostic outcome in both children and adults. t(1;19)(q23.3;p13.3) is another abnormality that is seen in approximately 5%

of children with pre-B-ALL. About 75% of patients show an unbalanced and 25% show a balanced form of this translocation, the unbalanced form in pediatric B-ALL patients is associated with a better prognostic outcome than the balanced form [62]. Three separate groups of hypodiploidy have been observed and are associated with an unfavorable prognosis. The most common is the near-haploid karyotype, with a chromosome count ranging from 26 to 29. The second is with chromosome count ranging from 30 to 39 and the third group with 40 to 44 chromosomes. Generally, a lower number of chromosomes correspond to a worse prognosis. Hyperdiploidy with chromosomes 51 and 55 is found to be associated with a relatively less favorable prognosis than those from 56 to 68 chromosomes. The presence of trisomies 4 and 10 are seemed to be with a better prognosis. The most common gains involve chromosomes 4, 6, 8, 10, 14, 17, 18, 19, and 21. The prognostic outcome of adult B-ALL patients with hyperdiploidy is not as favorable as in children. High hyperdiploidy is associated with poor prognosis [63–65]. Another abnormality often seen in children between 2 and 12 years old is the translocation t(12;21)(p13.2;q22.3) and is associated with a long duration of first remission and excellent cure rates. Another abnormality, del(9p) appears to be associated with improved outcomes in adults poor outcomes in children with B-ALL. Abnormalities like, dic(9;20)(p13.2;q11.2), dic(9;12) (p13.2;p12.2), and i(9)(q10), are associated with an excellent prognostic outcome. The most common rearrangements involving 14q32.3 observed in B-ALL are, t(8;14) (q11.2;q32.3), inv.(14)(q11.2q32.3), t(14;14)(q11.2;q32.3), t(14;19)(q32.3;q13.1), and t(14;20)(q32.3;q13.1) [64, 66, 67]. Approximately 10% of adults and 2% of children with B-ALL these translocations are more frequent. A rare translocation t(5;14)(q31.1;q32.3), has also been observed in B-ALL and is usually associated with eosinophilia. Other reported translocations are t(6;14)(p22.3;q32.3) and t(9;14)(p13.2;q32.3). Two cryptic translocations, t(X;14)(p22.3;q32.3) and t(Y;14) (p11.3;q32.3) have recently been described in B-ALL, especially in patients with Down syndrome. The abnormalities were usually seen in T-ALL involve 14q11.2, 7q35, 7p14. A rare but recurrent abnormality seen in T-ALL is inv. (14) (q11.2q32.1) or t(14;14) (q11.2;q32.1) [68–74].

3.2 Non-Hodgkin lymphoma (NHL)

NHL is a type of cancer that begins in the lymphatic system, comprises a heterogeneous group of disorders characterized by localized proliferation of lymphocytes. In non-Hodgkin's lymphoma, lymphocytes grow abnormally and can form tumors throughout the body. The most reliable criteria for the classification of malignant lymphomas are genetic abnormalities. The most common chromosome anomalies associated with specific lymphomas include t(14;18) (q32.3;q21.3) in follicular lymphoma (FL), t(8;14) (q24.2;q32.3) in Burkitt lymphoma (BL), t(11;14) (q13;q32.3) in mantle cell lymphoma (MCL), and t(11;18)(q21;q21.3) in mucosa-associated lymphoid tissue (MALT) lymphoma [75, 76].

3.3 Follicular lymphoma (FL)

FL is typically a slow-growing or indolent form of non-Hodgkin lymphoma (NHL) that arises from B-lymphocytes, making it a B-cell lymphoma. This lymphoma subtype accounts for 20–30% of all NHL cases. About 85–90% of patients with FL and 25–30% of patients with diffuse large B-cell lymphoma (DLBCL) exhibit (14;18)(q32.3;q21.3). Variant translocations, such as t(2;18)(p12;q21.3) and t(18;22)(q21.3;q11.2) have been described in both FL and DLBCL. Additional abnormalities in addition to t(14;18), certain numerical abnormalities, specifically trisomies 2, 7, and/or 8, are associated with a more favorable outcome.

Whereas patients with structural abnormalities, specifically del(1p), del(1q), del(6q), +der(18), or del(22q), or gain of an X chromosome or chromosome12, which are associated with an unfavorable outcome. Secondary abnormalities including +7, del(10q), del(6q), and/or +der(18) leads to the progression of FL to DLBCL occurs in 60–80% of cases [77–80].

3.4 Burkitt lymphoma (BL)

BL is a rare but highly aggressive B-cell NHL. This disease may affect the jaw, central nervous system, bowel, kidneys, ovaries, or other organs. Burkitt lymphoma may spread to the central nervous system (CNS). The most common abnormalities seen are t(8;14)(q24.2;q32.3), which is seen in about 75–80% of patients, t(8;22)(q24.2;q11.2) and t(2;8)(p12;q24.2), which are seen in 10% and 5% of patients, respectively [81, 82].

3.5 Diffuse large B-cell lymphoma (DLBCL)

DLBCL is the most common type of NHL, accounting for about 22% of newly diagnosed cases of B-cell NHL in the United States. In 25–30% of cases t(14;18)(q32.3;q21.3) is observed. Additional abnormalities seen are rearrangements of 1q and 3q, del(6q), +7, +8, del(10q), del(11q), +12, del(13q), rearrangements of 14q and 17p, +der(18)t(14;18), and +X. The more complex the karyotype the worse the prognostic outcome. Translocations involving 3q27 are found in approximately 35% of patients. More than 30 different partner genes have been translocated with this locus, the most recurrent of which include 2p12, 3q29, 4p13, 6p21.2, 6p22, 7p12, 8q24.2, 11q23, 13q14, 14q32.3, 15q22, 16p13, 17q11.2, 18p11.2, and 22q11.2. Other recurrent abnormalities observed are partial or complete gain of chromosome 3, specifically 3q; loss of chromosome 6; and gain of chromosome 18 and t(14;15)(q32.2;q11.2). Among these abnormalities, the only gain of chromosome 3 is associated with an adverse prognosis [83–88].

3.6 Mantle cell lymphoma (MCL)

MCL is typically an aggressive, rare form of NHL, in which about 95% of patients exhibit t(11;14)(q13;q32.3). t(2;11)(p12;q13), t(11;22) (q13;q11.2)], have been observed in a limited number of cases, but their detection is equally important for the diagnosis of MCL. t(12;14)(p13;q32;3), t(6;14)(p21;q32.3), t(2;14)(p24;q32.3), partial or complete gain of chromosomes 3 and 8, gain of 15q, and losses of 1p, 8p, 9p, 11q, 13q, loss of 9p, 17p, and gain of 3q and 8q, have also been described in MCL [89–92].

3.7 Mucosa-associated lymphoid tissue (MALT) lymphoma

This is a slow-growing type of non-Hodgkin lymphoma and, it most commonly develops in the stomach (when it is called gastric MALT lymphoma) but it can develop in other parts of the body also (which is called non-gastric MALT lymphoma). t(11;18)(q21.3;q21.3) is one of the specific chromosome aberrations occurring in 50% of MALT lymphoma cases. When present, this translocation is usually the only chromosome abnormality. The other specific translocation is (14;18)(q32.3;q21.3), which is observed in about 2% of cases. Abnormalities like, t(1;14)(p22.3;q32.3) and its variant t(1;2) (p22.3;p12 and t(3;14)(p13;q32.2) are also been observed [93–95].

3.8 Lymphoplasmacytic lymphoma (LPL)

This disorder presents with symptoms related to bone marrow infiltration and IgM monoclonal gammopathy. In approximately 50% of LPL cases, the deletion of 6q is observed, followed by a gain of chromosome 4 in 20% of cases, and abnormalities such as del(17p) and gains of chromosomes 3 and 7 in the small number of cases. The prognostic significance of chromosome abnormalities is unclear [96].

3.9 Splenic marginal zone B-cell lymphoma [SMZL]

SMZL represents a rare chronic B lymphocyte proliferative disease, which only accounts for about 1–2% of non-Hodgkin's lymphoma. Recurrent numerical and structural abnormalities are observed in SMZL. Deletion of 7q is one of the most common structural abnormalities, which is seen in approximately 30–40% of cases. In 30–50% of cases partial or complete trisomy 3 is seen and in 20–30% of cases partial or complete trisomy, 12 is observed. Deletion of 17p is seen in some aggressive cases in addition to these abnormalities [97–100].

3.10 Chronic lymphocytic leukemia (CLL)

CLL is an indolent B-cell neoplasm that leads to the proliferation of mature, normal-appearing lymphocytes in the peripheral blood, bone marrow, spleen, and lymph nodes. This is a type of non-Hodgkin lymphoma. The most important risk factor for the development of CLL is a positive family history. The prognosis is highly dependent on the presence of recurrent chromosome abnormalities, specifically del(6)(q23.3), del(13q)(q14.3), +12, del(11)(q22.1), and del(17)(p13.1) [101]. The presence of del(13q) is a sole abnormality and is considered as having a good prognosis. The deleted portion of chromosome 13 can vary in size, but it always involves band 13q14.3. Trisomy 12 is considered the second most common abnormality in CLL. Additional abnormality del (13q) is seen along with the gain of chromosome 12 in most cases and less frequently, del(11q) and del(17p), believed to occur mostly as clonal evolution. The presence of +12 together with del(14q) or t(14;18) has also been reported [102–105]. Deletion of 17p is another abnormality associated with loss of *TP53* at 17p13.1, are characterized by a poor response to chemotherapy and short survival. The majority of abnormalities leading to del(17p) are unbalanced translocations. Generally, the loss of 17p is present in the context of a complex karyotype. However, a few cases with i(17)(q10) as the only change have been described. Deletion of 6q is rarely the sole abnormality and this abnormality is considered an intermediate marker in CLL. Translocations involved chromosome 14 observed in CLL include t(11;14)(q13.q32.3), t(2;14)(p16.1;q32.3), t(14;19)(q32.3;q13), and t(14;18)(q32.3;q21.3), and their variants [105–110]. Rarely, t(8;14)(q24.2;q11.2) is observed as an additional abnormality in some CLL cases. Another recurrent translocation found to involve chromosome 13 is t(6;13)(p21;q14.1) or t(10;13)(q24;q14) [111, 112].

3.11 B-cell prolymphocytic leukemia

B-cell prolymphocytic leukemia (B-PLL) is a rare chronic lymphoproliferative neoplasm comprised of prolymphocytes, typically with involvement of the peripheral blood, bone marrow, and spleen, accounting for only 1% of all chronic leukemias of lymphoid origin. The important abnormalities reported are t(11;14), gain of chromosome 12, and deletions of 6q, 11q, 13q, and 17p, abnormalities. Additional abnormalities seen in some cases of PLL are the t(8;14), t(2;8), and t(8;22). In approximately 50% of cases, rearrangements of chromosome 17 leading to loss of 17p13.1 have been reported [113, 114].

3.12 Hairy cell leukemia (HCL)

HCL is a rare slow-growing B-cell lymphoproliferative neoplasm that accounts for 2% of all B-cell lymphomas. This affects more men than women, and it occurs most commonly in middle-aged or older adults. There are no specific chromosome abnormalities in HCL. However, a recurrent gain of chromosome 5, specifically the region 5q13-q31, and deletion of chromosome 7, specifically the region 7q22-q36 are demonstrated by conventional cytogenetics. Abnormalities involve chromosomes 1, 6, 14, and 19 are less frequently observed [115, 116].

3.13 Multiple myeloma (MM)

Multiple myeloma accounts for approximately 12% of hematologic neoplasms. This affects the terminally differentiated plasma cells in the bone marrow and presents with an excess of plasma cells in the bone marrow [117]. Chromosome abnormalities have been crucial in the characterization of prognostically significant markers in MM. Hypodiploidy (<46 chromosomes) with loss of chromosome 13, or chromosome 17, are associated with an unfavorable prognosis. In the majority of cases, the hypodiploid chromosome complement includes structural abnormalities, involving, in particular, chromosomes 1, 4, 6, 14, 16, and 20. Specifically, loss of 1p and/or gain of 1q, losses of 4q and 6q, loss and/or rearrangements of 14q and 16q, and partial or complete loss of chromosome 20 are most commonly seen. Translocations involving chromosome 14, are seen in approximately 85% of the cases, which include translocations, t(4;14)(p16.3;q32.3), t(14;16)(q32.3;q23.1), and t(14;20) (q32.3;q12) which are associated with an unfavorable prognosis. Karyotypes with 70–90 chromosomes and a double content of structural rearrangements, including the relative losses of chromosomes 13 and 17, most likely represent the doubling of a hypodiploid clone. Another group of MM patients is characterized by hyperdiploidy and few or no structural abnormalities. Gains are nonrandom and often involve chromosomes 3, 5, 7, 9, 11, 15, 19, and 21. Patients with the presence of these additional chromosomes are placed in a standard-risk category, as long as there is no deletion of 13q or 17p. The most common translocation in MM is t(11:14)(q13;q32.3) and is present in approximately 25% of cases and is associated with improved prognostic outcomes. The prognostic relevance of hyperdiploid karyotypes might be difficult to ascertain when structural abnormalities are present. An interstitial deletion of 13q, involving either 13q14.2 or 13q14.3, is one of the most common abnormalities in MM and has been detected in over 50% of cases. When other abnormalities present along with del(13q) appears to be with a poor prognosis. The prognostic outcome of a hyperdiploid karyotype typically associated with standard-risk myeloma is not altered by the presence of del(13q). On the other hand, in a hypodiploid karyotype, del(13q) or loss of chromosome 13 shows a poor prognosis. In approximately 10% of MM patients deletion of 17p has been observed which leads to deletion of 17p13.1 (*TP53*) and is believed that it occurs as secondary events during disease progression. This deletion is seen in both hypodiploid and hyperdiploid karyotypes. Contrary to what is seen with deletion of 13q, deletion of *TP53* has a negative impact, irrespective of the presence of favorable prognostic markers. Abnormalities involving chromosome 1 in MM include deletions of 1p, gains of 1q, and/or translocations involving either arm.

Deletions of 1p most frequently involve the segment between bands 1p12 and 1p31, whereas gain of 1q involves the segment q21 → qter or the entire long arm. Gain of 1q is the second most frequent chromosomal abnormality seen after del(13q). Among the translocations involving chromosome 1, the majority are derivatives of rearrangements involving various chromosomes, resulting in a gain of 1q. The common recurrent unbalanced translocations leading to gain of 1q are der(1;15)(q10;q10), der(1;16)(q10;p10), and der(1;19) (q10;p10). The most frequent non-random chromosomal partners found in translocations with 14q32.3, are t(11;14)(q13;q32.3), t(4;14)(p16.3;q32.3), and t(14;16)(q32.3;q23.1). t(11;14), is detected in about 20–25%, t(4;14)(p16.3;q32.3) is detected in approximately 15% and t(14;16)(q32.3;q23.1) is observed in approximately 5–7% of MM patients. Similarly to t(4;14), tends to occur in hypodiploid karyotypes, together with deletions of 13q and/or 17p, and this abnormality is placed in a high-risk prognostic category. Two other translocations, t(6;14)(p21.1;q32.3) and t(14;20) (q32.3;q12), have also been described in MM [118–126].

3.14 Hodgkin lymphoma (HL)

HL comprises approximately 30% of all lymphoma cases. HL affects individuals of all age groups with two preferential peaks, one occurring between the ages of 15 and 30 years and the other at 60 years. The majority of HL patients show a normal karyotype, abnormal chromosome complement is found in a minority of cases. There are no specific chromosome abnormalities been detected in HL. The common finding is that the karyotypes tend to be hyperdiploid, with 60–70 chromosomes. There are some recurrent abnormalities which include losses of 1p, 6q, 7q, 13q, 16q, and 17p; gains of 2p, 9p, and chromosome 12, as well as rearrangements of 3q27 [127, 128].

3.15 T-cell prolymphocytic leukemia (T-PLL)

T-PLL is a rare aggressive malignancy with poor response to conventional treatment and short survival. This affects approximately 2% of adults aged 30 years and over. The most common sites of involvement include peripheral blood, bone marrow, lymph node, and other hematopoietic organs such as the spleen and liver. T-PLL is with distinctive clinical, morphologic, and cytogenetic features. The most common chromosome abnormalities are inv.(14)(q11.2q32.1), t(14;14)(q11.2;q32.1), and t(7;14) (q34;q32.1). The most common translocation in this group is t(X;14)(q28;q11.2). In the majority of cases, additional abnormalities are observed, which include i(8)(q10) or other rearrangements leading to gain of 8q, deletion or rearrangements of 11q, and deletions of 6q, 12p, and 17p [129–131].

3.16 Adult T-cell leukemia/lymphoma (ATLL)

ATLL is a rare and often aggressive T cell Lymphoma that can be found in the blood (Leukemia), lymph nodes (Lymphoma), skin, or multiple areas of the body. Very complex karyotypes are observed in ATLL patients. The most frequent abnormalities include rearrangements of 7p14.1, 7q34, and 14q11.2; gains of the X chromosomes and chromosomes 3 and 7; rearrangements of 1p, 1q, 2q, 3q, and 17q; and deletions of 6q, 9p, 13q, and 17p. The prognosis associated with these abnormalities is considered an unfavorable prognosis. Abnormalities of 1p, 1q, 3q, and 14q and deletions of 2q, 9p, 14q, and 17p are found to be associated with poor prognosis [132–135].

3.17 Peripheral T-cell lymphoma, not otherwise specified (PTCL, NOS)

PTCL, NOS is a broad category of biologically and clinically heterogeneous diseases that cannot be further classified into any other of the existing entities defined by the WHO classification. Highly complex Karyotypes are usually seen with rearrangements that often lead to losses of 6q, 9p, 10q,13q and gains of 3q, 7q, and 8q and the prognosis is considered as poor for most patients. The t(5;9)(q33.3;q22.2) is an important translocation seen in these lymphomas [136, 137].

3.18 Angioimmunoblastic T-cell lymphoma (AITL)

AITL is a rare aggressive form of Non-Hodgkin's lymphoma which is a group of related malignancies. This accounts for approximately 2% of all non-Hodgkin's lymphomas but represents the most common subtype (15–20%) of peripheral T-cell lymphomas. Complex Karyotypes are seen and often show a gain of 11q13 and gains of chromosomes 3, 5, and an X chromosome, as well as losses of 5q, 10q, and 12q. Gain of 11q13 may represent a primary event in angioimmunoblastic T-cell lymphoma [138].

3.19 Anaplastic large cell lymphoma (ALCL)

ALCL is a rare type of NHL and is one of the subtypes of T cell Lymphoma ALCL comprises about 1% of all NHLs and approximately 16% of all T cell lymphomas [127]. The cytogenetic hallmark is the presence of specific translocations involving the anaplastic lymphoma kinase gene (ALK*)* and various partner chromosomes. The most common *ALK* translocation is t(2;5)(p23.1;q35.1), which fuses part of the nucleophosmin gene (*NPM1*) located at 5q35.1 with *ALK* located at 2p23.1, leading to activation of *ALK* [139, 140].

Author details

Hariharan Sreedharan
Division of Cancer Research, Regional Cancer Centre, Thiruvananthapuram, Kerala, India

*Address all correspondence to: shhrcc@gmail.com; shhrcc@rediffmail.com

References

[1] Taylor J, Xiao W, Abdel-Wahab O. Diagnosis and classification of haematologic malignancies on the basis of genetics. Blood. 2017;**130**(4):410-423

[2] Meloni-Ehrig A. Cytogenetic analysis. In: Body Fluid Analysis for Cellular Composition; Approved Guideline (H56A). Wayne: Clinical and Laboratory Standards Institute; 2006

[3] Gargallo P, Cacchione R, Chena C, et al. Chronic lymphocytic leukemia developing in a patient with chronic myeloid leukemia: Evidence of distinct lineage-associated genomic events. Cancer Genetics and Cytogenetics. 2005;**161**:74-77

[4] Robak T, Urbańska-Ryś H, Smolewski P, et al. Chronic myelomonocytic leukemia coexisting with B-cell chronic lymphocytic leukemia. Leukemia & Lymphoma. 2003;**44**(11):2001-2008

[5] Swerdlow SH, Campo E, Harris NL, et al. WHO Classification of Tumors of Haematopoietic and Lymphoid Tissues. Lyon: IARC; 2008

[6] Raskind WH, Tirumali N, Jacobson R, et al. Evidence for a multistep pathogenesis of myelodysplastic anemia. Blood. 1984;**63**:1318

[7] Bernasconi P, Boni M, Cavigliano PM, et al. Clinical relevance of cytogenetics in myelodysplastic syndrome. Annals of the New York Academy of Sciences. 2006;**1089**:395

[8] Olney HJ, Le Beau MM. Evaluation of recurring cytogenetic abnormalities in the treatment of myelodysplastic syndromes. Leukemia Research. 2007;**31**:427

[9] Sole F, Luno E, Sanzo C, et al. Identification of novel cytogenetic markers with prognostic significance in a series of 968 patients with primary myelodysplastic syndromes. Haematologica. 2005;**90**:1168

[10] Bacher U, Haferlach T, Kern W, et al. Conventional cytogenetics of myeloproliferative diseases other than CML contributes valid information. Annals of Hematology. 2005;**84**:250

[11] Mitelman F, Johansson B, Mertens F, editors: Mitelman Database of Chromosome Aberrations in Cancer [Internet]. 2008. Available from: http://cgap.nci.nih.gov/Chromosomes/Mitelman

[12] Bloomfield CD, Archer KJ, Mrozek K, et al. 11q23 balanced chromosome aberrations in treatment-related myelodysplastic syndromes and acute leukemia: Report from an international workshop. Genes, Chromosomes & Cancer. 2002;**33**:362

[13] Navada SC, Chatalbash A, Silverman LR. Clinical significance of cytogenetic manifestations in myelodysplastic syndromes. Laboratory Medicine. 2013;**44**:103-107

[14] Xu W, Li JY, Liu Q, et al. Multiplex fluorescence in situ hybridization in identifying chromosome involvement of complex karyotypes in de novo myelodysplastic syndromes and acute myeloid leukemia. International Journal of Laboratory Hematology. 2010; **32**:86-95

[15] Fialkow PJ, Jacobson RJ, Papayannopoulou T. Chronic myelocytic leukemia. Clonal origin in a stem cell common to the granulocyte, erythrocyte, platelet and monocyte/macrophage. The American Journal of Medicine. 1977;**63**:125

[16] Perrotti D, Jamieson C, Goldman J, Skorski T. Chronic myeloid leukemia:

Mechanisms of blastic transformation. The Journal of Clinical Investigation. 2010;**120**:2254-2264

[17] Nowell PC, Hungerford DA. A minute chromosome in human chronic granulocytic leukemia. Science. 1960;**132**:1497

[18] Rowley JD. A new consistent chromosomal abnormality in chronic myelogenous leukemia identified by quinacrine fluorescence and Giemsa staining. Nature. 1973;**243**:290

[19] Nacheva E, Holloway VT, Brown K, et al. Philadelphia negative chronic myelogenous leukemia: Detection by FISH of BCR-ABL fusion gene localized either to chromosome 9 or chromosome 22. British Journal of Haematology. 1993;**87**:409

[20] Karbasian Esfahani M, Morris EL, Dutcher JP, Wiernik PH. Blastic phase of chronic myelogenous leukemia. Current Treatment Options in Oncology. 2006; **7**:189-199

[21] Clark RE, Apperley JF, Copland M, et al. Additional chromosome abnormalities at chronic myeloid leukemia diagnosis predict an increased risk of progression. Blood Advances. 2021;**5**:4

[22] Adamson JW, Fialkow PJ, Murphy S, et al. Polycythemia vera: Stem cell and probable clonal origin of the disease. The New England Journal of Medicine. 1976;**295**:913

[23] Andrieux J, Demory JL. Karyotype and molecular cytogenetics studies in polycythemia vera. Current Hematology Reports. 2005;**4**:224

[24] Tang G, Hidalgo Lopez JE, Wang SA, et al. Characteristics and clinical significance of cytogenetic abnormalities in polycythemia vera. Haematologica. 2017;**102**:1511-1518. DOI: 10.3324/haematol.2017.165795

[25] Passamonti F, Rumi E, Arcaini L, et al. Leukemic transformation of polycythemia vera: A single center study of 23 patients. Cancer. 2005; **104**:1032-1036

[26] Jacobson RJ, Salo A, Fialkow PJ. Agnogenic myeloid metaplasia. A clonal proliferation of hematopoietic stem cells with secondary myelofibrosis. Blood. 1978;**51**:189

[27] Strasser-Weippl K, Steurer M, Kees M, et al. Prognostic relevance of cytogenetics determined by fluorescent in situ hybridization in patients having myelofibrosis with myeloid metaplasia. Cancer. 2006;**107**:2801

[28] Sever M, Kantarjian H, Pierce S, et al. Cytogenetic abnormalities in essential thrombocythemia at presentation and transformation. International Journal of Hematology. 2009;**90**:522-525

[29] Alvarez-Twose I, González de Olano D, Sánchez-Muñoz L, et al. Clinical, biological, and molecular characteristics of clonal mast cell disorders presenting with systemic mast cell activation symptoms. The Journal of Allergy and Clinical Immunology. 2010;**125**:1269-1278

[30] Brockow K, Metcalfe DD. Mastocytosis. Chemical Immunology and Allergy. 2010;**95**:110-124

[31] Elliott MA. Chronic neutrophilic leukemia and chronic myelomonocytic leukemia: WHO defined. Best Practice & Research. Clinical Haematology. 2006;**19**:571-593

[32] Orazi A, Cattoretti G, Sozzi G. A case of chronic neutrophilic leukemia with trisomy 8. Acta Haematologica. 1989;**81**:148-151

[33] Bowen DT. Chronic myelomonocytic leukemia: Lost in classification? Hematological Oncology. 2005;**23**:26-33

[34] Patnaik MM, Tefferi A. Cytogenetic and molecular abnormalities in Chronic myelomonocytic leukemia. Blood Cancer Journal. 2016;**6**:e393

[35] Pinheiro RF, MdeL C, Silva MR. Isochromosome 17q in MDS: A marker of a distinct entity. Cancer Genetics and Cytogenetics. 2006;**166**:189-190

[36] Tefferi A, Skoda R, Vardiman JW. Myeloproliferative neoplasms: Contemporary diagnosis using histology and genetics. Nature Reviews. Clinical Oncology. 2009;**6**:627-637

[37] Hasle H, Arico M, Basso G, et al. European Working Group on MDS in Childhood (EWOG-MDS). Myelodysplastic syndrome, juvenile myelomonocytic leukemia, and acute myeloid leukemia associated with complete or partial monosomy 7. Leukemia. 1999;**13**:376-385

[38] Betz BL, Hess JL. Acute myeloid leukemia diagnosis in the 21st century. Archives of Pathology & Laboratory Medicine. 2010;**134**:1427-1433

[39] Kantarjian H, Kadia T, DiNardo C, et al. Acute myeloid leukemia: Current progress and future directions. Blood Cancer Journal. 2021;**1**:41. DOI: 10.1038/s41408-021-00425-3

[40] Arber DA, Brunning RD, Le Beau MM, et al. Acute Myeloid Leukaemia and Related Precursor Neoplasms. WHO Classification of Tumours of Haematopoietic and Lymphoid Tissues. Revised 4th ed. Vol. 130. Lyon, France: IARC Press; 2017. p. 71

[41] Bendari M, Khoubila N, Cherkaoui S, et al. Current Cytogenetic Abnormalities in Acute Myeloid Leukemia. Vol. 10. Rijeka: IntechOpen; 2020. p. 5772

[42] Zhang Y, Le Beau MM. Cytogenetic abnormalities in acute myeloid leukemia. Up To Date. 2021

[43] Vakiti A, Mewawalla P. Acute Myeloid Leukemia, NCBI Bookshelf. A service of the National Library of Medicine, National Institutes of Health. Stat Pearls [Internet]. Treasure Island (FL): StatPearls Publishing; 2021

[44] Igarashi T, Shimizu S, Morishita K, et al. myelogenous leukemia with monosomy 7, inv(3)(q21q26), involving activated EVI 1 gene occurring after a complete remission of lymphoblastic lymphoma: A case report. Japanese Journal of Clinical Oncology. 1998; **28**:688-695

[45] Arber DA, Orazi A, Hasserjian R, et al. The 2016 revision to the World Health Organization classification of myeloid neoplasms and acute leukemia. Blood. 2016;**03**:643544

[46] Dastugue N, Lafage-Pochitaloff M, Pages MP, et al. Cytogenetic profile of childhood and adult megakaryoblastic leukemia (M7): A study of the Groupe Francais de Cytogenetique Hematologique (GFCH). Blood. 2002;**15**:618

[47] Seok JH, Park J, Kim SK, Choi JE, Kim CC. Granulocytic sarcoma of the spine: MRI and clinical review. AJR. American Journal of Roentgenology. 2010;**194**:485-489

[48] Zhang XH, Zhang R, Li Y. Granulocytic sarcoma of abdomen in acute myeloid leukemia patient with inv(16) and t(6;17) abnormal chromosome: Case report and review of literature. Leukemia Research. 2010; **34**:958-961

[49] Lee SG, Park TS, Cheong JW, et al. Preceding orbital granulocytic sarcoma in an adult patient with acute myelogenous leukemia with t(8;21): A case study and review of the literature. Cancer Genetics and Cytogenetics. 2008;**185**:51-54

[50] Douet-Guilbert N, Morel F, Le Bris MJ, et al. Rearrangement of MLL in

a patient with congenital acute monoblastic leukemia and granulocytic sarcoma associated with a t(1;11)(p36;q23) translocation. Leukemia & Lymphoma. 2005;**46**:143-146

[51] Marcus R, Sweetenham JW, Williams ME. Lymphoma: Pathology, Diagnosis and Treatment. Cambridge: Cambridge University Press; 2007. DOI: https://doi.org/10.1017/CBO9780511663369

[52] Steven H, Swerdlow EC, Pileri SA, et al. The 2016 revision of the world health Organization classification of Lymphoid neoplasms. The updated classification of haematological malignancies. Blood. 2016;**127**:20

[53] Pui C-H. Childhood Leukemias. 2nd ed. Vol. 2. New York: Cambridge University Press; 2006. pp. 774-804

[54] Faderl S, O'Brien S, Pui CH, et al. Adult acute lymphoblastic leukemia: Concepts and strategies. Cancer. 2010; **116**:1165-1176

[55] Roberts KG. Genetics and prognosis of ALL in children vs adults. Hematology American Society of Hematology. Education Program. 2018;**1**:137-145

[56] Szczepaõski T, Harrison CJ, van Dongen JJ. Genetic aberrations in paediatric acute leukaemias and implications for management of patients. The Lancet Oncology. 2010; **11**:880-889

[57] Ravandi F, Kebriaei P. Philadelphia chromosome-positive acute lymphoblastic leukemia. Hematology/Oncology Clinics of North America. 2009;**23**:1043-1063

[58] Zaccaria A, Testoni N, Valenti AM, et al. GIMEMA Working Party on CML. Chromosome abnormalities additional to the Philadelphia chromosome at the diagnosis of chronic myelogenous leukemia: Pathogenetic and prognostic implications. Cancer Genetics and Cytogenetics. 2010;**199**:76-80

[59] Wetzler M, Dodge RK, Mrózek K, et al. Additional cytogenetic abnormalities in adults with Philadelphia chromosome-positive acute lymphoblastic leukaemia: A study of the Cancer and Leukaemia Group B. British Journal of Haematology. 2004; **124**:275-288

[60] Fu JF, Liang DC, Shih LY. Analysis of acute leukemias with MLL/ENL fusion transcripts: Identification of two novel breakpoints in ENL. American Journal of Clinical Pathology. 2007; **127**:24-30

[61] De Braekeleer E, Meyer C, Le Bris MJ, et al. Identification of a MLL-MLLT4 fusion gene resulting from a t(6;11)(q27;q23) presenting as a del(11q) in a child with T-cell acute lymphoblastic leukemia. Leukemia & Lymphoma. 2010;**51**:1570-1573

[62] Forestier E, Johansson B, Gustafsson G, et al. Prognostic impact of karyotypic findings in childhood acute lymphoblastic leukaemia: A Nordic series comparing two treatment periods. For the Nordic Society of Paediatric Haematology and Oncology (NOPHO) Leukaemia Cytogenetic Study Group. British Journal of Haematology. 2000;**110**:147-153

[63] Harrison CJ, Moorman AV, Broad Field ZJ, et al. Childhood and Adult Leukaemia Working Parties. Three distinct subgroups of hypodiploidy in acute lymphoblastic leukaemia. British Journal of Haematology. 2004; **125**:552-559

[64] Zhang Y, Le Beau MM, Aster JC, et al. Classification, cytogenetics, and molecular genetics of acute lymphoblastic leukemia/lymphoma, all topics are updated as new evidence. www.uptodate.com © UpToDate. 2021

[65] Paulsson K, Johansson B. High hyperdiploid childhood acute lymphoblastic leukemia. Genes, Chromosomes & Cancer. 2009;**48**: 637-660

[66] Leblanc T, Derré J, Flexor M, et al. FISH analysis of translocations involving the short arm of chromosome 9 in lymphoid malignancies. Genes, Chromosomes & Cancer. 1997; **19**:273-277

[67] Heerema NA, Maben KD, Bernstein J, et al. Dicentric (9;20) (p11;q11) identified by fluorescence in situ hybridization in four pediatric acute lymphoblastic leukemia patients. Cancer Genetics and Cytogenetics. 1996;**92**:111-115

[68] Baumgarten E, Wegner RD, Fengler R, et al. Calla-positive acute leukaemia with t(5q;14q) translocation and hypereosinophilia—A unique entity? Acta Haematologica. 1989; **82**:85-90

[69] Russell LJ, Akasaka T, Majid A, et al. t(6;14)(p22;q32): A new recurrent IGH@ translocation involving ID4 in B-cell precursor acute lymphoblastic leukemia (BCP-ALL). Blood. 2008; **111**:387-391

[70] Iida S, Rao PH, Ueda R, et al. Chromosomal rearrangements of the PAX-5 locus in lymphoplasmacytic lymphoma with t(9;14)(p13;q32). Leukemia & Lymphoma. 1999;**34**:25

[71] MCA C, CNB A, JGC R, et al. Cytogenetic and molecular findings in children with acute lymphoblastic leukemia: Experience of a single institution in Argentina. Molecular Syndromology. 2015;**6**:193-203

[72] Hakeem A, Shiekh AA, Bhat GM, Lone AR. Prognostication of ALL by Cytogenetics. Indian Journal of Blood Transfusion. 2015;**31**(3):322-331

[73] Onciu M, Lai R, Vega F, et al. Precursor T-cell acute lymphoblastic leukemia in adults: Age-related immunophenotypic, cytogenetic, and molecular subsets. American Journal of Clinical Pathology. 2002;**117**:252-258

[74] Przybylski GK, Dik WA, Wanzeck J, Grabarczyk P, et al. Disruption of the BCL11B gene through inv(14) (q11.2q32.31) results in the expression of BCL11B-TRDC fusion transcripts and is associated with the absence of wild-type BCL11B transcripts in T-ALL. Leukemia. 2005;**19**(2):201-208

[75] Ma ESK. Recurrent cytogenetic abnormalities in non-hodgkin's lymphoma and chronic lymphocytic leukemia. Methods in Molecular Biology. 2017;**1541**:279-293. DOI: 10.1007/978-1-4939-6703-2_22

[76] Tri RL, Dunja MK, et al. Recurrent chromosome abnormalities in lymphomas in fine needle aspirates of lymph node. Collegium Anthropologicum. 2010;**2**:387-393

[77] Carbone A, Roulland S, Gloghini A, et al. Follicular lymphoma. Nature Reviews Disease Primers. 2019;**5**:83

[78] Jager U, Bocskor S, Le T, et al. Follicular lymphomas' BCL-2/IGH junctions contain templated nucleotide insertions: Novel insights into the mechanism of t(14;18) translocation. Blood. 2000;**95**:3520

[79] Bentley G, Palutke M, Mohamed AN. Variant t(14;18) in malignant lymphoma: A report of seven cases. Cancer Genetics and Cytogenetics. 2005;**157**:12-17

[80] Nanjangud G, Rao PH, Teruya-Feldstein J, et al. Molecular cytogenetic analysis of follicular lymphoma (FL) provides detailed characterization of chromosomal instability associated with the t(14;18) (q32;q21) positive and negative subsets

and histologic progression. Cytogenetic and Genome Research. 2007; **118**:337-344

[81] Stanley Maloy Kelly Hughes. Brenner's Encyclopedia of Genetics 2nd Edition. Academic Press. 2013: 4368

[82] Sietse M, Aukema LT, Rohde M, et al. Sequential karyotyping in Burkitt lymphoma reveals a linear clonal evolution with increase in karyotype complexity and a high frequency of recurrent secondary aberrations. British Journal of Hematology. 2015; **170**:814-825

[83] Susanibar-Adaniya S. Update on Diffuse large B cell lymphoma: A review of current data and potential applications on risk stratification and management. American Journal of Hematology. 2021;**96**:5

[84] Barrans SL, Evans PA, O'Connor SJ, et al. The t(14;18) is associated with germinal center derived diffuse large B-cell lymphoma and is a strong predictor of outcome. Clinical Cancer Research. 2003;**9**:2133-2139

[85] Abdel-Ghaffar H, El-Aziz SA, Shahin D, et al. Prognostic value of the t(14;18)(q32;q21) in patients with diffuse large B-cell lymphoma. Cancer Investigation. 2010;**28**:376-380

[86] Kim SY, Kim HJ, Kang HJ, et al. Clinical significance of cytogenetic aberrations in bone marrow of patients with diffuse large B-cell lymphoma: Prognostic significance and relevance to histologic involvement. Journal of Hematology & Oncology. 2013;**6**:76

[87] Barrans SL, O'Conner SJM, Evans PAS, et al. Rearrangement of the BCL6 locus at 3q27 is an independent poor prognostic factor in nodal diffuse large B-cell lymphoma. British Journal of Haematology. 2002;**117**:322

[88] Carbone A, Pantanowitz L, Sulfaro S, Gloghini A. B-cell lymphoma, unclassifiable, with features intermediate between diffuse large B-cell lymphoma and classical Hodgkin lymphoma. Atlas of Genetics Cytogenetics Oncolology Haematology. 2017;**21**(4):156-159

[89] Bertoni F, Zucca F, Cotter FE. Molecular basis of mantle cell lymphoma. British Journal of Haematology. 2004;**124**:130

[90] Li J-Y, Gaillard F, Moreau A, et al. Detection of translocation t(11;14)(q13;q32) in mantle cell lymphoma by fluorescence in situ hybridization. The American Journal of Pathology. 1999;**154**:1449

[91] Onciu M, Schlette E, Medeiros LJ, et al. Cytogenetic findings in mantle cell lymphoma cases with a high level of peripheral blood involvement have a distinct pattern of abnormalities. American Journal of Clinical Pathology. 2001;**116**:886-892

[92] Wlodarska I, Dierickx D, Vanhentenrijk V, et al. Translocations targeting CCND2, CCND3, and MYCN do occur in t(11;14)-negative mantle cell lymphomas. Blood. 2008;**111**:5683-5690

[93] Zullo A, Hassan C, Cristofari F, Perri F, Morini S. Gastric low grade mucosal-associated lymphoid tissue-lymphoma: *Helicobacter pylori* and beyond. World J Gastrointestinal Oncology. 2010;**2**:181-186

[94] Eric B. Staros: Different chromosomal translocations in MALT lymphoma promote cancer through a common mechanism. Laboratory Medicine. 2010;**41**(6):334-337

[95] Murga Penas EM, Callet-Bauchu E, Ye H, et al. The t(14;18)(q32;q21)/IGH-MALT1 translocation in MALT lymphomas contains templated nucleotide insertions and a major breakpoint region similar to follicular and mantle cell lymphoma. Blood. 2010;**115**:2214-2219

[96] Kern W, Haferlach T, Schnittger S, et al. Cytogenetic aberrations in lymphoplasmacytic lymphoma (lpl): A study on 166 cases. Blood. 2010;**116**:21

[97] Vallisa D, Bernuzzi P, Arcaini L, et al. Role of anti-hepatitis C virus (HCV) treatment in HCV-related, low-grade, B-cell, non-Hodgkin's lymphoma: A multicenter Italian experience. Journal of Clinical Oncology. 2005;**23**:468-473

[98] Baró C, Salido M, Espinet B, et al. New chromosomal alterations in a series of 23 splenic marginal zone lymphoma patients revealed by spectral karyotyping (SKY). Leukemia Research. 2008;**32**:727-736

[99] Gazzo S, Baseggio L, Coignet L, et al. Cytogenetic and molecular delineation of a region of chromosome 3q commonly gained in marginal zone B-cell lymphoma. Haematologica. 2003;**88**:31-38

[100] Brynes RK, Almaguer PD, Leathery KE, et al. Numerical cytogenetic abnormalities of chromosomes 3, 7, and 12 in marginal zone B-cell lymphomas. Modern Pathology. 1996;**9**:995-1000

[101] Baliakas SP, Jeromin S, Bartha K, Stamatopoulos K. Cytogenetic complexity in chronic lymphocytic leukemia: Definitions, associations, and clinical impact. Blood. 2019; **133**(11):1205-1216

[102] Tsimberidou AM, O'Brien S, Khouri I, et al. Clinical outcomes and prognostic factors in patients with Richter's syndrome treated with chemotherapy or chemoimmunotherapy with or without stem-cell transplantation. Journal of Clinical Oncology. 2006;**24**:2343-2351

[103] Calin GA, Dumitru CD, Shimizu M, et al. Frequent deletions and down-regulation of micro-RNA genes miR15 and miR16 at 13q14 in chronic lymphocytic leukemia. Proceedings of the National Academy of Sciences USA. 2002;**99**:15524-15529

[104] Van Dyke DL, Shanafelt TD, Call TG, et al. A comprehensive evaluation of the prognostic significance of 13q deletions in patients with B-chronic lymphocytic leukaemia. British Journal of Haematology. 2010; **148**:544-550

[105] Döhner H, Stilgenbauer S, Döhner K, et al. Chromosome aberrations in B-cell chronic lymphocytic leukemia: Reassessment based on molecular cytogenetic analysis. Journal of Molecular Medicine. 1999; **77**(2):266-281

[106] Reindl L, Bacher U, Dicker F, et al. Biological and clinical characterization of recurrent 14q deletions in CLL and other mature B-cell neoplasms. British Journal of Haematology. 2010;**151**:25-36

[107] Sen F, Lai R, Albitar M. Chronic lymphocytic leukemia with t(14;18) and trisomy 12. Archives of Pathology & Laboratory Medicine. 2002; **126**:1543-1546

[108] De Angeli C, Gandini D, Cuneo A, et al. BCL-1 rearrangements and p53 mutations in atypical chronic lymphocytic leukemia with t(11;14) (q13;q32). Haematologica. 2000; **85**(9):913-921

[109] Yin CC, Lin KI, Ketterling RP, et al. Chronic lymphocytic leukemia with t(2;14)(p16;q32) involves the BCL11A and IgH genes and is associated with atypical morphologic features and unmutated IgVH genes. American Journal of Clinical Pathology. 2009; **131**:663-670

[110] Bagacean C, Le Dantec C, Berthou C, et al. Combining cytogenetic and epigenetic approaches in chronic lymphocytic leukemia improves prognosis prediction for patients with

isolated 13q deletion. Clinical Epigenetics. 2017;**9**:122

[111] Karakosta M, Voulgarelis M, Vlachadami I, Manola KN. Translocation (6;13)(p21;q14.1) as a rare nonrandom cytogenetic abnormality in chronic lymphocytic leukemia. Cancer Genetics and Cytogenetics. 2010; **198**:66-70

[112] Baliakas P, Jeromin S, Iskas M, et al. Cytogenetic complexity in chronic lymphocytic leukemia: Definitions, associations, and clinical impact. Blood. 2019;**133**:1205-1216

[113] Gersen SL, Keagle MB, The Principles of Clinical Cytogenetics, Third Edition, © Springer Science+Business Media New York. 2013. DOI: 10.1007/978-1-4419-1688-4_15

[114] Chapiro E, Pramil E, Diop M'b, et al. Genetic characterization of B-cell prolymphocytic leukemia: A prognostic model involving MYC and TP53. Blood. 2019;**134**:1821-1831

[115] Solé F, Woessner S, Florensa L, et al. Cytogenetic findings in five patients with hairy cell leukemia. Cancer Genetics and Cytogenetics. 1999; **110**:41-43

[116] Vallianatou K, Brito-Babapulle V, Matutes E, et al. p53 gene deletion and trisomy 12 in hairy cell leukemia and its variant. Leukemia Research. 1999; **23**:1041-1045

[117] Palumbo A, Anderson K. Multiple myeloma. The New England Journal of Medicine. 2011;**364**:1046-1060

[118] Sawyer JR. The prognostic significance of cytogenetics and molecular profiling in multiple myeloma. Cancer Genetics. 2011; **204**:3-12

[119] Smadja NV, Bastard C, Brigaudeau C, et al. Hypodiploidy is a major prognostic factor in multiple myeloma. Blood. 2001;**98**:2229-2238

[120] Fonseca R, Barlogie B, Bataille R, et al. Genetics and cytogenetics of multiple myeloma: A workshop report. Cancer Research. 2004;**64**:1546-1558

[121] Zojer N, Koningsberg R, Ackermann J, et al. Deletion of 13q14 remains an independent adverse prognostic variable in multiple myeloma despite its frequent detection by interphase fluorescence in situ hybridization. Blood. 2000;**95**:1925

[122] Gertz MA, Lacy MQ, Dispenzieri A, et al. Clinical implications of t(11;14)(q13;q32), t(4;14)(p16.3;q32) and −17p13 in myeloma patients treated with high-dose therapy. Blood. 2005;**106**:2837

[123] Nadine Abdallah S, Rajkumar V, Greipp P, et al. Cytogenetic abnormalities in multiple myeloma: Association with disease characteristics and treatment response. Blood Cancer Journal. 2020;**10**:82

[124] Goldman-Mazur S, Vesole DH, Jurczyszyn A. Clinical implications of cytogenetic and molecular aberrations in multiple myeloma. Acta Haematologica Polonica. 2021;**52**:18-28

[125] Nishida K, Yashige H, Maekawa T, et al. Chromosome rearrangement, t(6;14) (p21.1;q32.3), in multiple myeloma. British Journal of Haematology. 1989;**71**:295-296

[126] Ross FM, Chiecchio L, Dagrada G, et al. The t(14;20) is a poor prognostic factor in myeloma but is associated with long-term stable disease in monoclonal gammopathies of undetermined significance. Haematologica. 2010;**95**:1221-1225

[127] Ma ESK. Recurrent cytogenetic abnormalities in non-hodgkin's lymphoma and chronic lymphocytic

leukemia. Cancer Cytogenetics. Methods in Molecular Biology. 2017;**1541**:279-293. DOI: 10.1007/978-1-4939-6703-2_22

[128] Wang H-W, Balakrishna JP, Pittaluga S, et al. Diagnosis of Hodgkin lymphoma in the modern era. British Journal of Haematology. 2019;**184**:45-59

[129] Colon Ramos A, Tarekegn K, Aujla A, et al. T-cell prolymphocytic leukemia: An overview of current and future approaches. Cureus. 2021;**13**(2): e13237. DOI: 10.7759/cureus.13237

[130] de Oliveira FM, Tone LG, Simões BP, Rego EM, et al. Translocations t(X;14)(q28;q11) and t(Y;14)(q12;q11) in T-cell prolymphocytic leukemia. International Journal of Laboratory Hematology. 2009;**31**:453-456

[131] Urbánková H, Holzerová M, Balcárková J, et al. Array comparative genomic hybridization in the detection of chromosomal abnormalities in T-cell prolymphocytic leukemia. Cancer Genetics and Cytogenetics. 2010; **202**:58-62

[132] Kamada N, Sakurai M, Miyamoto K, et al. Chromosome abnormalities in adult T-cell leukemia/lymphoma: A karyotype review committee report. Cancer Research. 1992;**52**:1481-1493

[133] Itoyama T, Chaganti RS, Yamada Y, et al. Cytogenetic analysis and clinical significance in adult T-cell leukemia/lymphoma: A study of 50 cases from the human T-cell leukemia virus type-1 endemic area, Nagasaki. Blood. 2001;**97**:3612-3620

[134] Sun Y, Murty VV, Leeman-Neill R, et al. Cytogenetic analysis of adult T-Cell leukemia/lymphoma: Evaluation of a Caribbean cohort. Leukemia & Lymphoma. 2019;**60**:1598-1600. DOI: 10.1080/10428194.2018.1538506

[135] Nakano N, Utsunomiya A, Matsuo K, et al. Chromosomal defects and survival in patients with adult T-cell leukemia/lymphoma after allogeneic HSCT. Blood Advances. 2021;**5**:475-486. DOI: 10.1182/bloodadvances.2020003639

[136] Lepretre S, Buchonnet G, Stamatoullas A, et al. Chromosome abnormalities in peripheral T-cell lymphoma. Cancer Genetics and Cytogenetics. 2000;**117**:71-79

[137] Jasmine M. Zain: Aggressive T-cell lymphomas: 2019 updates on diagnosis, risk stratification, and management. American Journal of Haematology. 2019;**94**:929-946

[138] Thorns C, Bastian B, Pinkel D, et al. Chromosomal aberrations in angioimmunoblastic T-cell lymphoma and peripheral T-cell lymphoma unspecified: A matrix-based CGH approach. Genes, Chromosomes & Cancer. 2007;**46**:37

[139] Perkins SL, Pickring D, Lowe EJ, et al. Childhood anaplastic large cell lymphoma has a high incidence of ALK gene rearrangements as determined by immunohistochemical staining and fluorescent in situ hybridization: A genetic and pathological correlation. British Journal of Haematology. 2005;**131**:624

[140] Zeng Y, Feldman AL. Genetics of anaplastic large cell lymphoma. Leukemia and Lymphoma. 2016; **57**:21-27

Chapter 8

Congenital Heart Disease and Surgical Outcome in Down Syndrome

Zainab Al-Suhaymi

Abstract

The prevalence of congenital heart disease has accounted for nearly one-third of all significant congenital anomalies worldwide. The first report about an association between cardiac anomalies and Down Syndrome was in (1876). Ten years after discovering of Down Syndrome and the credit of association between congenital cardiac anomalies and mongolism was suggested in (1894) by Garrod. There many studies performed to identify a correlation between genotype and phenotype in Down Syndrome, little is known about cardiovascular phenotype in Down Syndrome. Congenital heart disease is considered one of the highest causes of mortality and morbidity in Down Syndrome compared to patients with the same lesion of non-down. There is a big debate about surgical management and considered them as risk factors of surgery with precaution and recent technology, Down Syndrome considered as a normal patient in prognosis. This chapter aimed to shed the light on congenital heart disease in Down Syndrome and current knowledge in specific mutations associated with them and how the effect of innovative technology and management to treat them end at the same outcome and sometimes better based on recent research and Scoring System.

Keywords: Down Syndrome (DS), congenital heart disease (CHD), genetic mutations, surgical outcome, cardiovascular surgery

1. Introduction

1.1 History of congenital heart disease in Down Syndrome

Down Syndrome had a widespread revolutionary widespread interest since the days of Langdon Down's pioneering work in 1866 [1]. The first comprehensive description of this unique syndrome was provided in a short paper published in the London Hospital Reports [2]. Down's article was still unappreciated ten years later. In the July 1876 issue of the *Journal of Mental Science*, other reports on the same subject described the distinguishing features of an apparently new class of "idiots", and the first graphical illustration in the medical literature of DS was drawn in an article by Fraser and Mitchell. This also provided the first pictorial sketch of the facial features of a person with DS [3].

Awareness of DS medical reports was sketchy. It is almost incredible that DS was unknown before the last half of the nineteenth century [4]. In the 1960s,

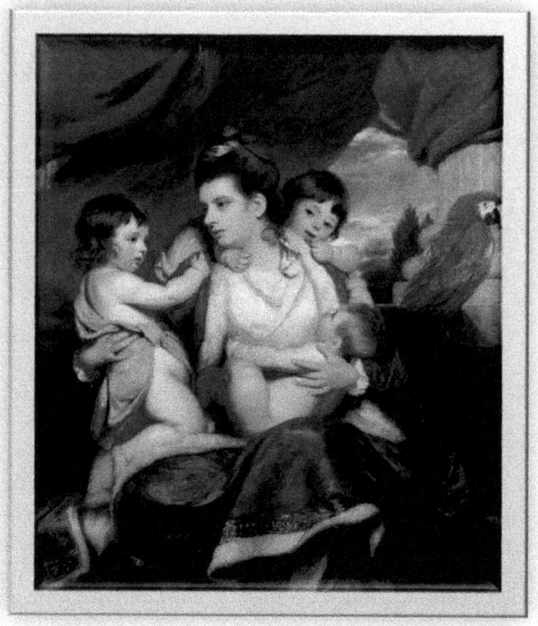

Figure 1.
The child looking over his mother's shoulder could be erroneously diagnosed as being affected with Down syndrome. Sir Joshua Reynolds's painting (1733) entitled Lady Cockburn and Her Children, which hangs in the National Gallery in London.

Iowa pediatrician Hans Zellweger was excited to find an illustration of a Down patient prior to the latter half of the nineteenth century **Figure 1**. A Down infant appeared in a painting by the Flemish artist Jacob Jordan entitled "Adoration of the Shepherds". This painting is dated 1618 and shows a woman holding a child (probably their daughter, Elizabeth) with similar DS features [5].

Other researchers have searched the art archives to determine pictorial representations of Down patients. In 1968, Dr. Arthur Markingson wrote a letter to the editor of Lancet in which he reported no painting of a Down patient could be found [6]. Dr. Markingson's letter prompted cogent reasons for the apparent rarity of Down children in past centuries. Populations were much smaller than they are now, and the population age structure was different only about two-thirds of females survived to the age at which they could marry. Only half reached the end of childbearing age. Infant mortality was also much higher.

In his opinion, this limited survival of infants with DS in history. In While there were fewer people, the rate of Down births would not have changed appreciably. This suggested that many Down children in the prior centuries did not survive the neonatal period. Thus, raises the question of why did they die? Many reasons must be considered. First, there were no modern therapies such as antibiotics and heart surgery. Down infants often die due to pulmonary infection and heart defects during the critical early years of life. CHD especially likely increased mortality [4–6].

2. Causative gene mutation

Congenital heart is a major public issue and health challenges. Understanding the molecular genetic mechanism underlying abnormal cardiac lesions associated with trisomy chromosome 21 may lead to novel therapies [7–10]. DS is the most common genetic causes of CHD and characterized by the presence of an extra full or partial human chromosome 21. In recent decades, significant efforts have been made to find the genotype-phenotype correlations for CHD in DS (DS CHD). For earlier detection and prevention and discover a better treatment.

There were several approaches to this problem: generating of a map of partial trisomy (PT21) cases in humans, creating mouse models with different orthologous regions of Hsa21, and analysis of DS gene expression in cells and tissues [11, 12]. Recent studies support the idea that not all Hsa21 loci are required for DS manifestation, suggesting a small region on 21q22.13 is considered critical to the DS core phenotype [13].

A primary goal of genetic studies in DS is to define sub-genomic areas associated with various DS phenotypes. There have been some exciting developments in this area after systematic analysis of 125 subjects from 1973 to 2015 (Pellerin et al., 2016). Retrospective reanalysis of the same cases added seven new topics (Piovesan et al., 2019) [13]. This work built a final map genomic region and discovered 34-kb on the distal part of 21q22.13 highly restricted DS critical region (HR-DSCR). Unfortunately, some patients carried additional chromosomal anomalies which makes the interpretation of genotype-phenotype correlation, including heart defects more difficult. Because of these complications, mice have been used instead of human partial (segmental) Ts21.

The long arm of Hsa21 has 33.9 Mega base in length and contains 430 protein-coding genes; 293 have a homolog in the mouse genome, and only 235 genes are conserved in syntonically regions on mouse chromosomes: (1) 16 (Mmu16, 23.3 Mb, 166 genes), (2) 17 (Mmu17, 1.1 Mb, 22 genes), and (3) 10 (Mmu10, 2.3 Mb, 47 genes). We found that Mmu16 is the only mouse chromosome associated with heart defects in DS [14, 15].

Mouse models associated with congenital heart disease are shown in **Figure 2**. The first is the Tc1 mouse model, which carries Hsa21, where approximately 8% of its genes were deleted leading to heart defects [16, 17]. The second is Ts65D, which is the most widely used model [18]. And exhibits some major DS phenotypes, including heart defects [19, 20]; Ts65Dn is trismic for 13.4 Mb of the 22.9 Mb Hsa21 syntenic region on Mmu16. The cardiovascular phenotype of overlapping in larger-than-5.8 Mb sub-centromeric region on Mmu17, which is not syntactic to any region on Hsa21 [21].

We recently developed new rodent models to understand and mimic DS mouse segmental trisomy. The third type of model is Dp (10)1Yey/+, Dp (16)1Yey/+ and

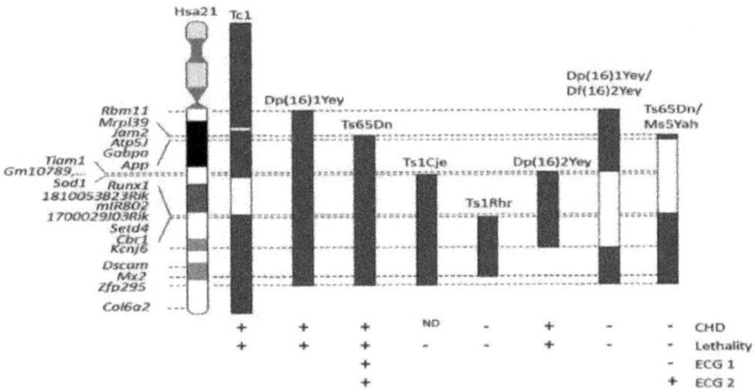

Figure 2.
Representation of the DS mouse models associated with cardiac features. "+" indicates the presence and "-" the absence of phenotypes whereas ND indicates a non-determined state for presence or absence of CHD in Ts1Cje.

Dp (17)1Yey/+, carrying individual duplications spanning the entire Hsa21 syntenic regions on Mmu10, Mmu16, and Mmu17, respectively. The results showed both Dp (16)1Yey/+Dp (10)1Yey/+; Dp (16)1Yey/+; and Dp (17)1Yey/+ contribute to heart defects with similar frequency. The final model showed heart defect in Dp (16)2Yey/+ embryos within the Tiam1-Kcnj6 region correlated with over-expression of 20 genes in this area [22].

CHD in DS is a phenotype characterized by reducing the extent to which a particular gene or set of genes expressed in the phenotypes of individuals carrying it. Consequently, in PT21 cases mapping, it is possible to exclude chromosomal regions or identify them as critical for the phenotype only in patients with that phenotype (DS CHD). Approaching the DS CHD critical region was proposed by Korenberg et al. [23] when his concept used the 9 Mb region between D21S55 (21q22.2) to the telomere for the first time. This work further used mouse models over 4–5 Mb region, from (D21S55 through MX1) Korbel et al. [24] narrowed down the critical part for DS CHD to 1.77 Mb, **Figure 3**. The region in question was extended from DSCAM to ZNF295 (current name ZBTB21) created from combining the maps of 14 PT21 subjects with CHD with information from segmental trisomic mouse model Dp (16)1Yu/+.

In 40–60% of subjects, the overall risk of DSCHD in DS is from AVSDs [25]. Although some candidate genes have been a cause for DSCHD, conclusive evidence for their involvement is still unknown. We previously reported a map that contains the DSCHD region in humans to a 5.27-Mb chromosomal segment containing 82 genes [26]. **Figure 3A** narrows down this segment to a 2.82-Mb critical region likely involved in DSCHD endocardial cushion defects using an expanded panel with 14 subjects with DSCHD. By integrating our information from segmental trisomic mouse models with DSCHD [16, 21], we integrated a further limit on this region in a particular map (**Figure 3B**); we propose a 1.77-Mb DSCHD critical region, which contains ten genes, including the promoter and a portion of the DS cell adhesion molecule (DSCAM) gene. Specifically, the model Dp (16)1Yu/shows that DSCHD is involved only in the HSA21 regions orthologous to MMU16 (located at 14.4 Mb–42.3 Mb of HSA21); this defines the telomeric DSCHD border and suggests a limited role for the adjacent telomeric region for DSCHD.

2.1 Genes associated with causing CHD

A multifactorial model used as sample collection. Chromosome 21 Single nucleotide polymorphisms calling and Chromosome 21 Copy number variations analyses by pyrosequencing and Sanger sequencing showed most notable results of this study regarding identifying CHD risk loci in DS [27].

1. rs2832616 and rs1943950 are CHD risk alleles (odds ratios of 2.8 and 2.7, respectively) within the same LD block on chromosome 21 (both cis-eQTLs for KRTAP7–1 gene).

2. A 4.9-kb CNV upstream of the RIPK4 gene (CNV1) the RIPK4 gene (CNV1) has a risk ratio of 2.29 in the previously reported CHD region of chromosome 21.

3. A 1.8-kb CNV within the ZBTB21 gene (CNV2) of chromosome 21 with a risk ratio of 1.85. in the previously reported CHD region.

4. A pair of interacting cis-eQTLs on chromosome 11 (Bonferroni-adjusted P-value <0.05). involving CNOT11 on chromosome 2 and NRGN.

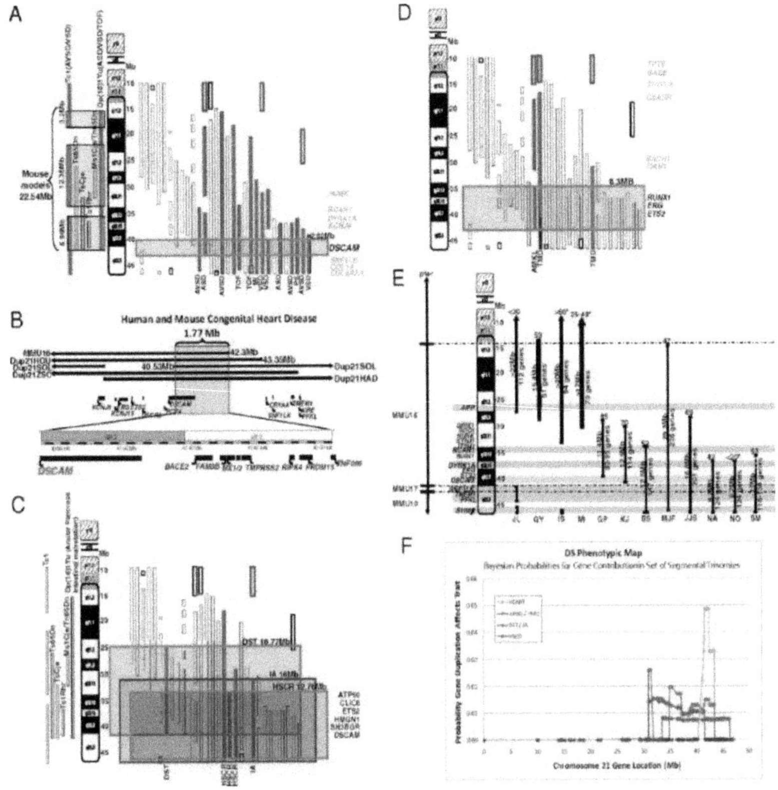

Figure 3.
A panel of 30 patients with segmental trisomy 21 metanalysis defines DS phenotype candidate regions. Yellow boxes, no phenotype; solid boxes, increased copy-number; open boxes, 1:2 (monosomies) Purple boxes, presence of phenotype. (A) DSCHD region. TOF, tetralogy of Fallot; PS, pulmonic stenosis; PDA, patent ductus arteriosus; VSD, ventricular septal defect; ASD, atrial septal defect; MI, mitral insufficiency. Red box, DSCHD candidate region. Twenty-three subjects have duplications, including the DSCHD region, 14 thereof have DSCHD. No subject lacking a segmental trisomy involving the DSCHD critical regions was diagnosed with DSCHD. Corresponding regions for six mouse models are indicated to the left [21, 22, 39–41]. (B) Proposed DSCHD critical region (red box) determined by combining human and mouse data from A. MMU16 indicates the extent of the duplication in the mouse model Dp (16)1Yu with DSCHD.

3. Clinical management

3.1 Diagnostic evaluation

Echocardiograms are generally accepted as the diagnostic standard. Some studies specified that all had an echocardiogram [49], while others limited by documentation and relied on retrospective review [28]. One study evaluated if screening, chest X-ray and ECG is an effective method to identify which infants with DS should have an echocardiogram. They found that this method resulted in 69 (17%) fewer echocardiograms without missing infants with major CHD [29]. A similar study showed a sensitivity of 71% and a specificity of 91% chest X-ray and ECG soon after birth for three modalities separately or in combination to detect CHD [30].

3.2 Surgical approach

DS is a challenging public health issue. The survival rate of DS with heart defects has increased dramatically with improved medical care [31]. Infant mortality for patients with DS remain 5× to 8× higher than that of the general population. In the 1940s to 1960s, the average life expectancy for children born with DS dramatically increased from 12 years in the 1940s to 60 [32]. There has been a gradual improvement in the results of DS children undergoing cardiac surgery in the last 16 years [33] with a better understanding of surgical anatomy, Advances in surgical techniques improved myocardial protection and cardiopulmonary bypass strategies, and advances in postoperative management in the intensive care unit contributed to improved survival rate and decreased mortality [34–36].

When comparing the DS to NS in preoperative data, however there are significant differences in age, RACHS-1 risk category, and presence of substantial noncardiac anomalies among DS patients in the 30 days (about four and a half weeks) to 1 year age group. In contrast, most children in the non-DS patients were in the >1 year age group. The DS population is more likely to have a coexisting major noncardiac structural anomaly, although DS were less likely to have been born prematurely [32].

In open-heart surgery, the cardiopulmonary bypass led to prolonged times. [(110 ± 47 min), 129 (87.75%), and (101.74 ± 33.61)]; aortic cross-clamp was shorter [(65 ± 30 min), 64 minutes (67.21 ± 26.63)]. Depend on the scoring system most patients in DS and Non-DS, RACHS-1 risk categories 1, 2, and 3. Distribution for patients without DS were spread across these three risk categories. In DS, the proportion of patients in risk categories 1, 2, and 3 increased with increasing surgical complexity [32, 37].

Infection is the most common complication that feared by surgeons and results in a more prolonged ICU and hospitalization with considerable treatment in patients with CHD and DS [38]; respiratory complications are also common. Sepsis occurred in 8 patients (10%), mainly caused by Staphylococcus and Pseudomonas. In 7/8 cases, this infection occurred early in the postoperative period. In one case, sepsis developed late and led to death [33].

4. Types of producers associated with DS

4.1 Favorable surgical outcome

4.1.1 Complete atrioventricular septal defect

Hospital mortality ranges from 0.9 to 3% in recent studies [39, 40]. The degree of residual valve dysfunction was independent of surgical choice in a study comparing three surgical techniques [41]. LV outflow tract obstruction is the second cause for reintervention small left ventricle (LV) and a double orifice left the atrioventricular valve. There was an anatomic increase in reoperation incidences, such as a small left ventricle (LV) and a double orifice left atrioventricular valve [41]. The hospital resources usage for cardiac surgery in pediatric patients with CHD and genetic conditions is of great interest [42]. Patients with DS and AVSD heart defect did not constitute an extra financial burden due to good surgical outcome and short hospital stay.

4.1.2 Partial atrioventricular septal defects

Mortality rate was low (0–1%) and reported with repair performed in early childhood [43]. The left atrioventricular valve anatomy was unfavorable in 31% of cases. Reoperation was required in 22% of non-DS. All patients survived surgery.

Other issues include:

4.1.3 single ventricle physiology and Unbalanced atrioventricular septal defects

There is often univentricular palliation or correction (Fontan-type) due to the constant risk of pulmonary hypertension or even mildly elevated pulmonary vascular resistance. Excellent survival was noted at palliation when pulmonary vascular resistance was low (<3 Wood Units/m2) in the 1st year of life. The mortality rate of patients with Fontan-type repair was 27.5% in patients with unbalanced AVSD [44]. Moreover, Fontan-type repair was rarely performed and was considered risky (12% early mortality) in Japan [45]. Furukawa et al. reported eight patients with Down syndrome who underwent total cardiopulmonary connection; one patient died, whereas the clinical course and recovery after surgery in the other seven patients was significantly prolonged. They studied 17 patients with DS who underwent TCPC and reported that mortality in the early period was 29% and significantly higher than that in patients without DS (10%). The debate is now DS itself is a vital independent factor of mortality. Future work should evaluate mortality and long-term prognosis.

4.2 Unfavorable surgical outcome

4.2.1 Tetralogy of Fallot

Cyanosis in DS patients accounts for about 6% of deaths. Early mortality has been reduced to 1–2% in recent years [39, 46, 47]; pulmonary hypertension is presumed to be a causal factor, and this was supported by its higher incidence in patients with tetralogy of Fallot associated with AVSD. Patients with DS and tetralogy of Fallot need a pulmonary valve replacement (PVR)/implantation earlier than normal patients [48].

4.2.2 Tetralogy of Fallot combined with AVCanal

This is a rare anomaly frequently associated with DS and low operative risk (4–6%) has been recently accomplished Complete repair [49] two-stage (with prior palliation) and single-stage repair was recently reported. With 10-year survival obtained the two strategies as well as similar freedom from reoperation for left atrioventricular valve regurgitation [50].

5. Scoring systems in cardiac surgical outcome

5.1 RACHS-score

The RACHS-1 method [51, 52] was used to adjust for differences in the patient mix when comparing in-hospital death. Surgical procedures ranged from 1 to 6 risk categories. Risk category 1 has the lowest risk for in-hospital death, whereas risk category 6 has the highest. Risk categories 5 and 6 were combined for reporting purposes because of the low numbers of patients in each group. Patients with >1 cardiac surgical procedure were placed in the category of the highest risk procedure.

Two studies evaluated outcomes in children with DS by grouping cardiac lesions based on risk-stratified categories (RACHS-1). There were generally low mortality rates for children with DS compared to those without, which highlighting the higher rate of cardiac operations in DS children [32, 39].

5.2 Aristotle score

A new international Nomenclature of evaluating the quality of care in congenital heart surgery based on the complexity of the surgical procedures the project started in 1999, involving expert surgeons included 50 pediatric surgeons from 23 countries representing International Scientific Societies. The calculation is undertaken in two steps: the first adjusts only the complexity of the procedures by establishing the Basic Score determined by three factors: the potential for morbidity, the anticipated technical difficulty, the potential for mortality. The second step was improving the Comprehensive Score, which further adjusts the complexity according to the specific patient characteristics. The Aristotle method allows the following equation of quality of care: Complexity FN Outcome = Performance which allows precise scoring of the complexity for 145 congenital heart surgery procedures. The complexity was based on the procedures defined by the Society of Thoracic Surgeons (STS)/European Association for Cardiothoracic Surgery (EACTS) [53].

5.3 Propensity score matching analysis

Propensity score matching was frequently used in the cardiovascular surgery literatures. These methods are increasingly used to reduce the impact of treatment-selection bias in estimating causal treatment effects using observational data [54–56]. Tóth et al. reported that the perioperative values had no significant differences between the DS and non-DS groups after propensity matching. This method used similar values for the variables and can play an essential role in identifying the differences between control and study groups.

In *Seminars in Thoracic and Cardiovascular Surgery,* the propensity score used at 5:1, (NS: DS). PSM based on sex, low birth weight, and prematurity age group with post matching standardized mean difference indicating successful balancing of the two groups; the final matched set was 2493 DS patients. These were compared to 12,465 patients, as shown in **Figure 4**.

We show outcomes after cardiac operations in patients with DS using Texas Inpatient Public Use Datafile was queried for all patients <18 years old undergoing

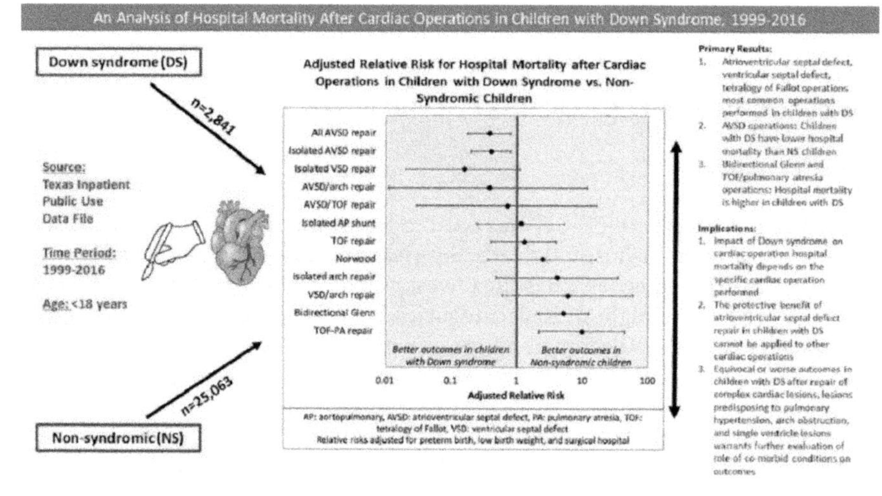

Figure 4.
Children with Down syndrome and non-syndromic children undergoing various cardiac operations represented by The Texas Inpatient Public Use Datafile was queried from 1999 to 2016.

CHD procedures between 1999 and 2016. There were 2,841 cases in DS patients who underwent CHD operations compared to 25,063 non-DS cases. Over the 18-year period. Variables depending on the type of CHD lesion when multiple cardiac lesions require intervention; DS children have an excellent surgical outcome and hospital survival after isolated AVSD than did non-DS children. Bidirectional Glenn palliation TOF/PA repair was associated with worse hospital mortality in children with DS. Further work will be evaluated cardiac and noncardiac comorbidities in DS patients led to higher mortality for specific cardiac lesions [57].

6. Conclusion

The challenge of cardiac care of DS patients has no more concerns because of a great improving result of cardiac surgery contribute to the increasing survival and to the better quality of life is even more successful and gratifying.

Conflict of interest

The authors declare no conflict of interest.

Author details

Zainab Al-Suhaymi
Resident General Surgery, General Surgery Department, Prince Mohammed Bin Abdul Aziz Hospital, Ministry of National Guard Health Affairs, Al-Madinah, Saudi Arabia

*Address all correspondence to: zainab.alsuhaymi@gmail.com

References

[1] M. C. Liu and K. Corlett, "A Study of Congenital Heart Defects in Mongolism," *Archives of Disease in Childhood* 34, no. 177 (October 1959): 410-19.

[2] "Langdon-Down-1866.Pdf," accessed February 21, 2021, https://www.romolocapuano.com/wp-content/uploads/2013/07/Langdon-Down-1866.pdf.

[3] FRASER J. Kalmuc idiocy: report of a case with autopsy with notes on 62 cases. Journal of Mental Science. 1876; 22:161.

[4] E. Peter Volpe, "Is Down Syndrome A Modern Disease" Perspectives in Biology and Medicine 29, no. 3 (1986): 423-36, https://doi.org/10.1353/pbm.1986.0043.

[5] H. W. HEFKE, "ROENTGENO LOGIC STUDY OF ANOMALIES OF THE HANDS IN ONE HUNDRED CASES OF MONGOLISM," American Journal of Diseases of Children 60, no. 6 (December 1, 1940): 1319-23, https://doi.org/10.1001/archpedi.1940.02000060077008.

[6] Mirkinson A. IS DOWN SYNDROME A MODERN DISEASE? The Lancet. 1968 Jul 13;292(7559):103.

[7] "EBSCOhost | 31851823 | Adult Congenital Heart Disease: A 2008 Overview.," accessed February 21, 2021, https://web.b.ebscohost.com/abstract?direct=true&profile=ehost&scope=site&authtype=crawler&jrnl=00071420&AN=31851823&h=A8qVAXqHvxOwiGv6GsBKq%2fe13NW%2fvf0BYb0JgeLceSjxGmXikChS8NtQKzVrfxJsjmEU92HUEsKT4NlNwzFyPQ%3d%3d&crl=c&resultNs=AdminWebAuth&resultLocal=ErrCrlNotAuth&crlhashurl=login.aspx%3fdirect%3dtrue%26profile%3dehost%26scope%3dsite%26authtype%3dcrawler%26jrnl%3d00071420%26AN%3d31851823.

[8] Priya Pillutla, Kanaka D. Shetty, and Elyse Foster, "Mortality Associated with Adult Congenital Heart Disease: Trends in the US Population from 1979 to 2005," American Heart Journal 158, no. 5 (November 1, 2009): 874-79, https://doi.org/10.1016/j.ahj.2009.08.014.

[9] Williams Roberta G. et al., "Report of the National Heart, Lung, and Blood Institute Working Group on Research in Adult Congenital Heart Disease," Journal of the American College of Cardiology 47, no. 4 (February 21, 2006): 701-7, https://doi.org/10.1016/j.jacc.2005.08.074.

[10] Ariane J. Marelli et al., "Planning the Specialized Care of Adult Congenital Heart Disease Patients: From Numbers to Guidelines; an Epidemiologic Approach," American Heart Journal 157, no. 1 (January 1, 2009): 1-8, https://doi.org/10.1016/j.ahj.2008.08.029.

[11] P. Aula, J. Leisti, and H. von Koskull, "Partial Trisomy 21," Clinical Genetics 4, no. 3 (1973): 241-51, https://doi.org/10.1111/j.1399-0004.1973.tb01149.x.

[12] Stylianos E. Antonarakis, "10 Years OfGenomics,Chromosome 21, and Down Syndrome," Genomics 51, no. 1 (July 1, 1998): 1-16, https://doi.org/10.1006/geno.1998.5335.

[13] Maria Chiara Pelleri et al., "Systematic Reanalysis of Partial Trisomy 21 Cases with or without Down Syndrome Suggests a Small Region on 21q22.13 as Critical to the Phenotype," Human Molecular Genetics, April 22, 2016, ddw116, https://doi.org/10.1093/hmg/ddw116.

[14] Odilkys Cala Hernández, "Caracterización Del Síndrome de Down En La Población Pediátrica," Revista de Ciencias Médicas de Pinar Del Río 17, no. 4 (August 2013): 33-43.

[15] Robert Lyle et al., "Genotype–Phenotype Correlations in Down Syndrome Identified by Array CGH in 30 Cases of Partial Trisomy and Partial Monosomy Chromosome 21," European Journal of Human Genetics 17, no. 4 (April 2009): 454-66, https://doi.org/10.1038/ejhg.2008.214.

[16] Aideen O'Doherty et al., "An Aneuploid Mouse Strain Carrying Human Chromosome 21 with Down Syndrome Phenotypes," Science 309, no. 5743 (September 23, 2005): 2033-37, https://doi.org/10.1126/science.1114535.

[17] D. A. Devenny et al., "Dementia of the Alzheimer's Type and Accelerated Aging in Down Syndrome," Science of Aging Knowledge Environment: SAGE KE 2005, no. 14 (April 6, 2005): dn1, https://doi.org/10.1126/sageke.2005.14.dn1.

[18] R. H. Reeves et al., "A Mouse Model for Down Syndrome Exhibits Learning and Behaviour Deficits," Nature Genetics 11, no. 2 (October 1995): 177-84, https://doi.org/10.1038/ng1095-177.

[19] Clara S. Moore, "Postnatal Lethality and Cardiac Anomalies in the Ts65Dn Down Syndrome Mouse Model," Mammalian Genome: Official Journal of the International Mammalian Genome Society 17, no. 10 (October 2006): 1005-12, https://doi.org/10.1007/s00335-006-0032-8.

[20] Adam Williams and Richard A. Flavell, "The Role of CTCF in Regulating Nuclear Organization," Journal of Experimental Medicine 205, no. 4 (March 17, 2008): 747-50, https://doi.org/10.1084/jem.20080066.

[21] Li Z, Yu T, Morishima M, Pao A, LaDuca J, Conroy J, et al. Duplication of the entire 22.9 Mb human chromosome 21 syntenic region on mouse chromosome 16 causes cardiovascular and gastrointestinal abnormalities. Hum Mol Genet. 2007 Jun 1;16(11):1359-66.

[22] Liu P, Zhang H, McLellan A, Vogel H, Bradley A. Embryonic Lethality and Tumorigenesis Caused by Segmental Aneuploidy on Mouse Chromosome 11. Genetics. 1998 Nov 1;150(3):1155-68.

[23] Korenberg JR, Chen XN, Schipper R, Sun Z, Gonsky R, Gerwehr S, et al. Down syndrome phenotypes: The consequences of chromosomal imbalance. PROC NAT ACAD OF SCI (USA). 1994 May 24;91(11):4997-5001.

[24] Jan O. Korbel et al., "The Genetic Architecture of Down Syndrome Phenotypes Revealed by High-Resolution Analysis of Human Segmental Trisomies," Proceedings of the National Academy of Sciences of the United States of America 106, no. 29 (July 21, 2009): 12031-36, https://doi.org/10.1073/pnas.0813248106.

[25] Claudine P. Torfs and Roberta E. Christianson, "Anomalies in Down Syndrome Individuals in a Large Population-Based Registry," American Journal of Medical Genetics 77, no. 5 (1998): 431-38, https://doi.org/10.1002/(SICI)1096-8628(19980605)77:5<431::AID-AJMG15>3.0.CO;2-J.

[26] G. M. Barlow et al., "Down Syndrome Congenital Heart Disease: A Narrowed Region and a Candidate Gene," Genetics in Medicine: Official Journal of the American College of Medical Genetics 3, no. 2 (April 2001): 91-101, https://doi.org/10.1097/00125817-200103000-00002.

[27] M. Reza Sailani et al., "The Complex SNP and CNV Genetic Architecture of the Increased Risk of Congenital Heart Defects in Down Syndrome," Genome Research 23, no. 9 (September 1, 2013):

1410-21, https://doi.org/10.1101/gr.147991.112.

[28] Echocardiogram [Internet]. nhs.uk. 2017 [cited 2021 Feb 21]. Available from: https://www.nhs.uk/conditions/echocardiogram/

[29] Bogarapu S, Pinto NM, Etheridge SP, Sheng X, Liesemer KN, Young PC, et al. Screening for Congenital Heart Disease in Infants with Down Syndrome: Is Universal Echocardiography Necessary Pediatr Cardiol. 2016 Oct 1;37(7):1222-7.

[30] Tubman TR, Shields MD, Craig BG, Mulholland HC, Nevin NC. Congenital heart disease in Down syndrome: two-year prospective early screening study. BMJ. 1991 Jun 15;302(6790):1425-7.

[31] Dimopoulos K, Kempny A. Patients with Down syndrome, and congenital heart disease: survival is improving, but challenges remain. Heart. 2016 Oct 1;102(19):1515-7.

[32] Evans JM, Dharmar M, Meierhenry E, Marcin JP, Raff GW. Association Between Down Syndrome and In-Hospital Death Among Children Undergoing Surgery for Congenital Heart Disease: A US Population-Based Study. Circ Cardiovasc Qual Outcomes. 2014 May;7(3):445-52.

[33] Kabbani MS, Giridhar S, Elbarbary M, Elgamal M-A, Najm H, Godman M. Postoperative cardiac intensive care outcome for Down syndrome children. Saudi Med J. 2005 Jun;26(6):943-6.

[34] Kobayashi M, Takahashi Y, Ando M. Ideal timing of surgical repair of isolated complete atrioventricular septal defect. Interactive CardioVascular and Thoracic Surgery. 2007 Feb 1;6(1):24-6.

[35] Yasui H, Nakamura Y, Kado H, Yonenaga K, Shiokawa Y, Fusazaki N, et al. Primary repair for complete atrioventricular canal: Recommendation for early primary repair. JCARDIOVASCSURG. 1990;31(4):498-504.

[36] Suzuki T, Bove EL, Devaney EJ, Ishizaka T, Goldberg CS, Hirsch JC, et al. Results of Definitive Repair of Complete Atrioventricular Septal Defect in Neonates and Infants. The Annals of Thoracic Surgery. 2008 Aug 1;86(2):596-602.

[37] Hoashi T, Hirahara N, Murakami A, Hirata Y, Ichikawa H, Kobayashi J, et al. Current Surgical Outcomes of Congenital Heart Surgery for Patients with Down Syndrome in Japan. Circ J. 2018;82(2):403-8.

[38] Santos FCGB, Croti UA, Marchi CHD, Murakami AN, Brachine JDP, Borim BC, et al. Surgical Treatment for Congenital Heart Defects in Down Syndrome Patients. Brazilian Journal of Cardiovascular Surgery. 2019 Feb;34(1):1-7.

[39] Fudge JC, Li S, Jaggers J, O'Brien SM, Peterson ED, Jacobs JP, et al. Congenital Heart Surgery Outcomes in Down Syndrome: Analysis of a National Clinical Database. PEDIATRICS. 2010 Aug 1;126(2):315-22.

[40] St. Louis JD, Jodhka U, Jacobs JP, He X, Hill KD, Pasquali SK, et al. Contemporary outcomes of complete atrioventricular septal defect repair: Analysis of the Society of Thoracic Surgeons Congenital Heart Surgery Database. The Journal of Thoracic and Cardiovascular Surgery. 2014 Dec 1;148(6):2526-31.

[41] Pontailler M, Kalfa D, Garcia E, Ly M, Le Bret E, Roussin R, et al. Reoperations for left atrioventricular valve dysfunction after repair of atrioventricular septal defect. European

Journal of Cardio-Thoracic Surgery. 2014 Mar 1;45(3):557-63.

[42] Furlong-Dillard J, Bailly D, Amula V, Wilkes J, Bratton S. Resource Use and Morbidities in Pediatric Cardiac Surgery Patients with Genetic Conditions. The Journal of Pediatrics. 2018 Feb 1; 193:139-146.e1.

[43] Bowman JL, Dearani JA, Burkhart HM, Goodloe AH, Phillips SD, Weaver AL, et al. Should Repair of Partial Atrioventricular Septal Defect Be Delayed Until Later in Childhood? The American Journal of Cardiology. 2014 Aug 1;114(3):463-7.

[44] Polimenakos AC, Subramanian S, ElZein C, Ilbawi MN. Attrition in patients with single ventricle and trisomy 21: outcomes after a total cavopulmonary connection. Interactive CardioVascular and Thoracic Surgery. 2017 May;24(5):747-54.

[45] Hoashi T, Hirahara N, Murakami A, Hirata Y, Ichikawa H, Kobayashi J, et al. Current Surgical Outcomes of Congenital Heart Surgery for Patients with Down Syndrome in Japan. Circ J. 2018;82(2):403-8.

[46] Dey S. Advances in Research on Down Syndrome. BoD – Books on Demand; 2018. 150 p.

[47] Sullivan RT, Frommelt PC, Hill GD. Earlier Pulmonary Valve Replacement in Down Syndrome Patients Following Tetralogy of Fallot Repair. Pediatr Cardiol. 2017 Aug 1;38(6):1251-6.

[48] Prifti E. Repair of complete atrioventricular septal defect with tetralogy of Fallot. Transl Pediatr. 2017 Jan;6(1):1-7.

[49] Vitanova K, Cleuziou J, Schreiber C, Günther T, Pabst von Ohain J, Hörer J, et al. Long-Term Outcome of Patients with Complete Atrioventricular Septal Defect Combined with the Tetralogy of Fallot: Staged Repair Is Not Inferior to Primary Repair. The Annals of Thoracic Surgery. 2017 Mar 1;103(3):876-80.

[50] Jenkins KJ, Gauvreau K, Newburger JW, Spray TL, Moller JH, Iezzoni LI. Consensus-based method for risk adjustment for surgery for congenital heart disease. The Journal of Thoracic and Cardiovascular Surgery. 2002 Jan 1;123(1):110-8.

[51] Jenkins KJ, Gauvreau K. Center-specific differences in mortality: Preliminary analyses using the Risk Adjustment in Congenital Heart Surgery (RACHS-1) method. The Journal of Thoracic and Cardiovascular Surgery. 2002 Jul 1;124(1):97-104.

[52] Jacobs JP, Jacobs ML, Lacour-Gayet FG, Jenkins KJ, Gauvreau K, Bacha E, et al. Stratification of Complexity Improves the Utility and Accuracy of Outcomes Analysis in a Multi-Institutional Congenital Heart Surgery Database: Application of the Risk Adjustment in Congenital Heart Surgery (RACHS-1) and Aristotle Systems in the Society of Thoracic Surgeons (STS) Congenital Heart Surgery Database. Pediatr Cardiol. 2009 Sep 23;30(8):1117.

[53] Lacour-Gayet F, Clarke D, Jacobs J, Gaynor W, Hamilton L, Jacobs M, et al. The Aristotle score for congenital heart surgery. Semin Thorac Cardiovasc Surg Pediatr Card Surg Annu. 2004;7:185-91.

[54] ROSENBAUM PR, RUBIN DB. The central role of the propensity score in observational studies for causal effects. Biometrika. 1983 Apr 1;70(1):41-55.

[55] Rosenbaum PR, Rubin DB. Reducing Bias in Observational Studies Using Subclassification on the Propensity Score. null. 1984 Sep 1;79(387):516-24.

[56] Grunkemeier GL, Payne N, Jin R, Handy JR. Propensity score analysis of stroke after off-pump coronary artery bypass grafting. The Annals of Thoracic Surgery. 2002 Aug 1;74(2):301-5.

[57] Dhillon GS, Ghanayem NS, Broda CR, Lalani SR, Mery CM, Shekerdemian LS, et al. An Analysis of Hospital Mortality After Cardiac Operations in Children With Down Syndrome. Seminars in Thoracic and Cardiovascular Surgery. 2020 Dec 1;32(4):947-57.

Section 5

Prenatal Screening, Management and Counseling in Down Syndrome and Other Chromosomal Abnormalities

Chapter 9

Prenatal Screening of Aneuploidies

Madhavilatha Routhu and Shiva Surya Varalakshmi Koneru

Abstract

Chromosomal abnormalities includes 1) abnormalities in number of chromosomes which are known as aneuploidies and 2) structural defects like translocations and deletions. In this we will discuss about Aneuploidies The incidence of Aneuploidy is around one in 200 live births. Aneuploidy increases with advancing maternal age. Fetal aneuploidy has been associated with significant pregnancy complications such as growth restriction, congenital malformations and perinatal deaths. Several Major developments are happened in prenatal screening of Aneuploidy especially the introduction of first trimester screen with Nuchal thickness and fetal cell free DNA in maternal plasma and identification of ultrasound markers and biochemical screening in second trimester. In this chapter we will discuss about what are trisomies, why "Down syndrome" is important to detect prenatally, history of "Down syndrome", advances in screening methods biochemical as well as sonographic markers in first and second trimester and the criteria to get those markers. What are the features of trisomy 21, trisomy18 and trisomy13.

Keywords: Aneuploidies 1, "Down syndrome" 2, ultrasound markers 3, Nuchal translucency 4

1. Introduction

Aneuploidies are Trisomy21 ("Down syndrome", T21), Trisomy18 (Edward syndrome, T18), trisomy13 (Patau syndrome, T13), monosomy (turner syndrome, monosomy) and triploidy. "Down syndrome" is more focused than other aneuploidy due to Trisomy 13 and 18 are lethal, do not have very long-term consequences, and almost all cases have major structural abnormalities and can be identified on the basis of these features. Where as in T21 the ultrasound and laboratory findings are subtle and nonspecific. Special effort has to be made to identify these nonspecific features and analyse their importance. Identification of T21 is based on these subtle abnormal structures i.e., ultrasound markers and abnormal biochemistry (low PAPP-A and raised β-HCG). The abortion rate in monosomy X is 98% and Edwards is 86% whereas "Down syndrome" is only 30%. Not only this Downs is the commonest congenital cause of mental disability with long life span and need life-long family support. The incidence is 1in 800 pregnancies. Downs can lead to considerable ill health, although some individual may have only mild problems and can lead relatively normal lives. Having baby with "Down syndrome" is likely to have significant impact on family life. There is currently no known cure. A significant number of parents would opt for terminating such a pregnancy or if they want to continue prior information would benefit for preparing for such a baby. Downs occur due to non-disjunction type (Errors in meiosis). Translocation type and mosaic type which is rare.

2. History

In 1862 & 1887 Langdon Down noted that common characteristics of patients with trisomy 21 are skin deficient in elasticity, giving the impression of being too large for the body, and face is flat, broad and destitute of prominence. The cheeks are roundish and extended laterally. The eyes are obliquely placed, and internal canthi more than normally distanced from one another. The palpebral fissure is very narrow. The tongue is long, thick and much roughened. The nose is small. In 1987 B Benacerraf [1], told that this loose skin can be seen in mid trimester scan at 20 weeks as a thickening of skin at the back of neck in axial view of skull in trans cerebellar plane which was defined as nuchal fold. After 5 years it was realized that the excess skin of individuals with Down's syndrome can be visualized by ultrasonography as increased nuchal translucency in the third month of intrauterine life [2]. About 75% of trisomy 21 fetuses have increased nuchal translucency (NT) and 60–70% have absent nasal bone.

2.1 History of screening methods

Aneuploidy increases with advancing maternal age. So, increasing the maternal age increases the risk. in the early 1970s, the screening was based only on the association with advanced maternal age. In late 1980s not only maternal age but also found that the concentration of various fetoplacental products in the maternal circulation has taken into account for screening. At 16 weeks of gestation the median maternal serum concentrations of alpha-fetoprotein (AFP), un-conjugated estriol (μE3), human chorionic gonadotropin (HCG) (free- β and total) and inhibin-A in aneuploidy are sufficiently different from normal to allow the use of combinations or some or all of these substances to select high risk group. This method is more effective than maternal age alone. It can identify about 60–70% of the fetuses with T21. In1990s, screening by a combination of maternal age and fetal NT thickness at 11–13 + 6 weeks of gestation was introduced. This method shown to identify about 75–80% of affected fetuses for a screen-positive rate of about 5%. There by,

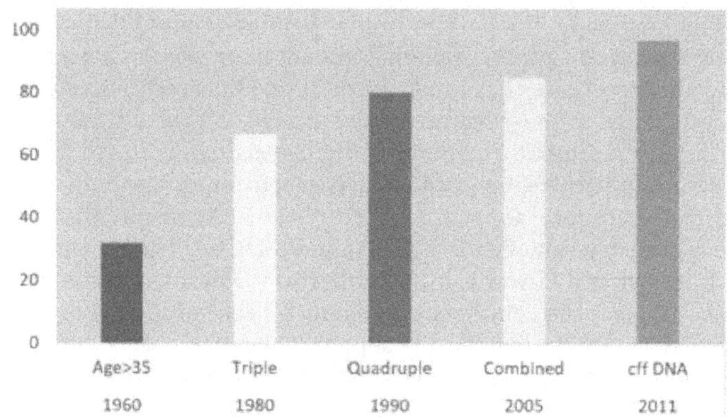

Figure 1.
Aneuploidy screening Approach: observed Detection rates.

maternal age was combined with fetal NT and maternal serum biochemistry (free β-HCG and PAPP-A) in the first-trimester to identify about 85–90% of affected fetuses. In 2001, it was found that 60–70% Trisomy 21 fetuses were associated with non-visualized nasal bone. Inclusion of nasal bone and the other ultrasound markers to NT and biochemistry for the screening procedure increase the detection rate in to more than 95% in first trimester with a screen positive rate of 2.5% (**Figure 1**). Furthermore, introduction of one-stop clinics for assessment of risk (OSCAR) which is a new method of biochemical testing, where with-in 30 min of taking blood sample, made it possible to assess the risk [3, 4].

3. Type of screening tests

"Down syndrome" can be diagnosed during pregnancy. Diagnostic tests are invasive and have an inherent miscarriage rate, however, small they are also expensive. Screening tests can identify a large number of patients who would benefit from diagnostic testing thus reducing risks and costs. Screening tests by definition, cannot identify all accepted pregnancies. First trimester screening is far more effective than later screening. Aneuploidy screening should be offered to all the pregnant women.

Screening tests that are performed in the first and second trimesters include integrated, sequential and contingent screening. The basic types are 1) first trimester combined screening the components in this are Nuchal translucency (NT), PAPP-A and β-HCG. The detection rate is 85–95%. If you add nasal bone and other ultrasound features to this the detection rate increases 93–96%. 2) Triple test the components are β-HCG, MS-AFP and unconjugated Estriol. The detection rate is only 60–65%. 3) Quadruple test β-HCG, MS-AFP, unconjugated Estriol and inhibin A. the detection rate is 70–75%. 4) Penta screen includes hyper glycosylated HCG in addition to quadruple test. If patient come for screening in first trimester, first trimester combined screening is advised, if she comes at 14-20 weeks quadruple test, if she comes at both first and second trimester integrated test is best for screening (**Table 1**).

Integrated test:-Integrate the First trimester PAPP-A, Free β-HCG and NT analyte screening followed by a second trimmester Quad screen and receives a single

Methods of screening	Detection rate	False-positive rate
Maternal age(MA)	30%	5%
First trimester		
MA+ fetal nuchal translucency(NT)	75–80%	5%
MA+ serum free β-hCG and PAPP-A	60–70%	5%
MA + NT + free β-hCG and PAPP-A (combined Test)	85–95%	5%
Combined Test+ nasal bone or tricuspid flow or ductus venosus flow	93–96%	2.5%
Second trimester		
MA + serum AFP,hCG, μE3(triple test)	60–65%	5%
MA + serum AFP,free β-hCG, μE3, inhibin A(Quadruple test)	70–75%	5%
MA + NT + PAPP-A(11-13 weeks) + quadruple test	90–94%	5%
Nicolaides KH. Screening for fetal aneuplodies at 11t013weeks.Prenat Diagn 2011;31:7–15.		

Table 1.
Methods of screening and its detection rate.

screen test result. The detection rate of this test is 90–94%. Limitations includes the withholding of first trimester screening test results until the second trimester which delay the management option.

Sequential screening: - these are two types one is stepwise another one is contingent model. These methods were developed to maintain a high detection rate. in step wise sequential model it can be achieved by using the combined first and second trimester screening approach while also reporting the patients first trimester screening test risk, which allows for earlier management options. If first trimester test result is higher than lab derived positive screening cutoff, we can offer them the diagnostic test or NIPT, and the screening protocol is discontinued. If the patient has a lower risk can counseled and proceed to quad screening in the second trimester. Sequential screening has a detection rate of 91–93% with a positive screening test result rate of 4–5% [5–7].

Contingent model classifies aneuploidy risk as high, intermediate or low on the basis of first trimester screening test results. High risk patients are offered cell free DNA screening or diagnostic testing with CVS and for low risk women further screening or testing is not recommended. Only those with intermediate risk are offered second trimester screening.

4. Method of sequential screening

Every woman has a risk that her fetus has a chromosomal abnormality.

4.1 Standard first trimester aneuploidy screening

to calculate the individual risk, the clinical information which is necessary to take into account the background or a priori risk, depends on maternal age, weight the ethnicity (in terms of south Asian, east Asian, south east Asian black or Caucasian), IVF, number of fetuses diabetes and smoking. This information should be combined with ultrasound information and biochemistry. Which is based on crown rump length, NT, PAPP-A, free β-HCG. Then make calculation by a series of factors or likelihood ratios, which depend on the results of a series of screening tests carried out during the course of the pregnancy to determine the patient-specific risk. A priori risk established by maternal age has been adjusted successfully by NT screening. This has been one of the most important elements of aneuploidy screening as it resulted in a significant reduction in unnecessary invasive testing on pregnant women with advanced maternal age. If you add rest of the ultrasound features like nasal bone, ductus venosus and tricuspid regurgitation which can increase the rate of detection.

4.2 Standard genetic sonogram aneuploidy screening

Genetic sonogram has been used to screen for Aneuploidy by using specific findings. In this approach seeks major structural abnormalities and minor ultrasonographic soft markers. These Soft markers are minor ultrasound abnormalities, considered as variants of normal, they do not constitute a structural defect. Presence of Soft markers are indicative of an increased age adjusted risk of an underlying fetal aneuploidy or some non- chromosomal abnormalities. So, these are also a priori risk. Detection of soft markers increase the risk for aneuploidy by constant proportion (likelihood ratio LR). Absence of these markers lower the risk (Negative predictive value NPV). These were decided after a meta-analysis study of second trimester markers for trisomy21 [8], (**Table 2**).

Marker	LR+(95%CI)	LR-(95%CI)	LR isolated marker*
Intra cardiac echogenic focus	5.83(5.02–6.77)	0.80(0.75–0.86)	0.95
Ventriculomegaly	27.52(13.61–55.68)	0.94(0.91–0.98)	3.81
Increased nuchal fold	23.30(14.35–37.83)	0.80(0.74–0.85)	3.79
Echogenic bowel	11.44(9.05–14.47)	0.90(0.86–0.94)	1.65
Mild Hydronephrosis	7.63(6.11–9.51)	0.92(0.89–0.96)	1.08
Short humerus	4.81(3.49–6.62)	0.74(0.63-o.88)	0.78
Short femur	3.72(2.79–4.97)	0.80(0.73–0.88)	0.61
ARSA	21.48(11.48–40.19)	0.71(0.57–0.88)	3.94
Absent or hypoplastic nasal bone	23.27(14.23–38.06)	0.46(0.36–0.58)	6.58

Table 2.
Meta-analysis of 2nd trimester markers for trisomy21-M. Agathokleous et al.

Every time a test is carried out the *a priori* risk is multiplied by *the likelihood ratio* of the test to calculate a new risk, which then becomes the *a priori* risk for the next test [9].

If a systematic second- trimester ultrasound examination demonstrates the absence of all major defects and markers, there is a 7.7fold reduction in risk for trisomy 21. Detection of any one of the markers during the scan should stimulate the sonographer to look for all other markers or defects. Post-test odds for trisomy 21 is derived by multiplying the pre-test odds by the positive LR for each detected marker and the negative LR for each marker demonstrated to be absent.

In Sequenitial screening first do the first trimester combined screening test identify the risk based on this risk if it is high risk do the invasive procedure (CVS) or NIPT. If there is false positive and false negetive results then you need to combine with quadraple test and sequentially calcuate the risk as the false positive rate is very very low.

5. Biochemical markers

First trimester markers are pregnancy associated plasma protein A (PAPP-A), Free β Human chorianic gonadotropin (β-HCG) where as second trimester markers are Alpha fetoprotein (AFP) Unconjugated oestriol (μE3), Total human chorianic gonadotropin (HCG) and inhibin-A.

The PAPP-A level is low in T21 which is about half of euploid pregnancies. β-HCG levels are double that of unaffected pregnancies. The concentrations of these markers vary with gestational age. In first trimester PAPP-A increases and free β-HCG decreases. In second trimester AFP and μE3 increase HCG and inhibin-A will decreases before 17 weeks after that it may increas. The measurements of these markers may vary between laboratories. In account of this variation the concentration of each marker is expressed as multiple of median for unaffected pregnancies of the same gestational age (MoM).

6. First trimester sonographic markers

provision of a high-quality first trimester screening service significantly enhances the autonomy of pregnant women [10].

6.1 Nuchal translucency (NT)

The gestation should be 11–13 + 6 weeks and the fetal crown–rump length should be 45–84 mm. Criteria for the Standardized Measurement of the Nuchal translucency at 11–13 + 6 weeks are- fetus must be in the midsagittal plane. The image must be magnified so, that it is filled by the fetal head, neck and upper thorax, the magnification should be as large as possible and each slight movement of the callipers should produce only a 0.1 mm change in the measurement. The fetal neck must be in neutral position, it should not be flexed, and not hyperextended. Amnion must be seen separate from NT line. The margins of NT edges must be clear enough for proper placement of the callipers (**Figure 2**). The + callipers on the ultrasound must be used to perform the NT measurement. Electronic callipers must be placed on the inner borders of the nuchal line space with none of the horizontal crossbar itself protruding into the space and the callipers must be placed perpendicular to the fetal long axis. Measurement must be obtained at the widest space of the NT. Cord round the neck may be present in 5–10% of cases which may produce a falsely increased NT. In such cases, the measurements of NT above and below the cord are different so, the average of these two measurements should be appropriate for calculating risk. One of the studies involving 96,127 pregnancies, at a crown rump length of 45 mm the median and 95th centile was 1.2 and 2.1 mm and the crown rump length of 84 mm were 1.9 and 2.7 mm [11]. The average NT in aneuploidy is about 2.5 mm above the normal median for crown-rump length. In Turner syndrome, the median NT is about 8 mm above the normal median.

6.2 Nasal bone (NB)

It may be present, absent or hypoplastic. In the normal fetus between the 11th and early 12th week of gestation, the nasal bone may appear poorly ossified or absent [12]. In such cases, it is recommended to repeat the measurement one week later [12]. Nasal bone hypoplasia is calculated as BPD/NBL ratio if >11 than hypoplasia. Several studies have demonstrated a high association between absent nasal bone at 11–13 + 6 weeks and trisomy 21, as well as other chromosomal abnormalities [13]. Criteria for the Standardized Measurement of the Nasal Bone at 11–13 + 6 weeks are mid sagittal view of face with the magnification of the image should be such that the fetal head and thorax occupy the whole screen. Mid sagittal face is defined by the presence of the echogenic tip of the nose and rectangular

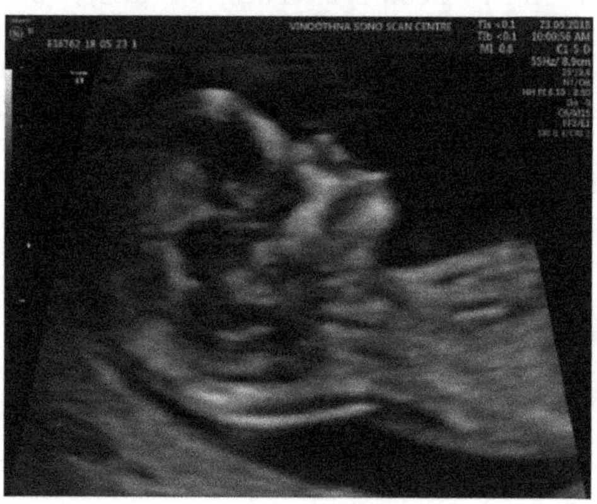

Figure 2.
Normal NT and nasal bone.

shape of the palate anteriorly, the translucent diencephalon in the center, and the nuchal membrane posteriorly. Minor deviations may cause non-visualization of the tip of the nose and visibility of the zygomatic process of the maxilla. The ultrasound transducer should be parallel to the direction of the nose and it should be gently tilted from side to side to ensure that the Nasal bone is seen separate from the skin (**Figure 2**). The echogenicity of NB should be greater than the overlying skin. Three distinct lines are noted in nasal bone demonstration: the first two lines are horizontal and parallel to each other where the top line represents the skin and bottom line is the NB. Third one represents the tip of the nose. When the NB line appears as a thin and less echogenic than the overlying skin, which suggests that the NB is not yet ossified, and it is classified as being absent (**Figure 5**) [12].

6.3 Ductus venosus (DV)

Criteria for the Standardized Measurement of DV at 11–13 + 6 weeks are the magnification of the image should be such that the fetal head and thorax should occupy the whole screen. Right ventral mid sagittal view of fetal trunk should be obtained. Color flow mapping of umbilical vein DV and fetal heart should be

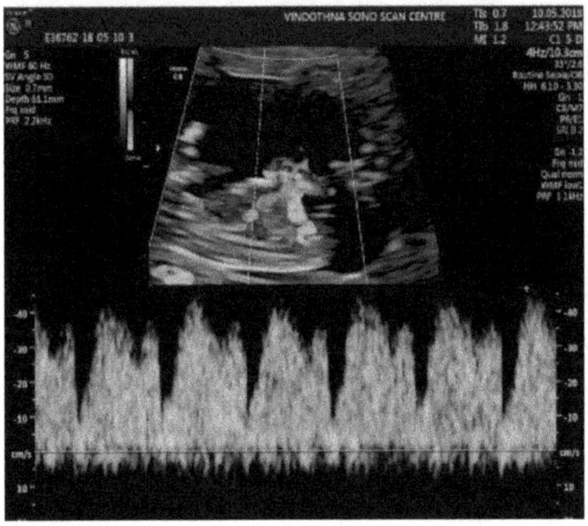

Figure 3.
Normal ductus venosus.

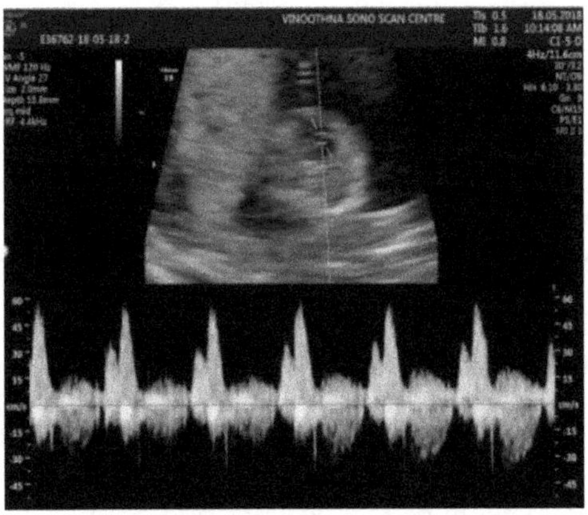

Figure 4.
Normal tricuspid valve.

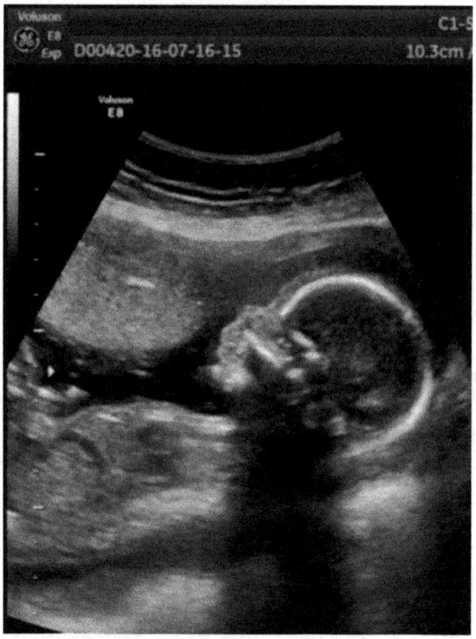

Figure 5.
Absent nasal bone.

demonstrated. Pulse doppler sample volume should be small (0.5–1.0 mm) and it should be placed in the yellowish aliasing area. Insonation angle should be less than 30degrees [12]. The filter should be set at a low frequency (50-70 Hz). Sweep speed should be high (2-3 cm/s) so that the waveforms are spread allowing better assessment of the A wave (**Figure 3**). Ductus venosus shows biphasic wave form with low pulsatility and antegrade flow in the diastolic components (a wave) throughout cardiac cycle. Normal ductus venosus Doppler waveforms show a positive a-wave, whereas the presence of an absent or reversed a-wave defines abnormal ductus venosus waveforms. The presence of high pulsatility or reverse flow of the a-wave in the first trimester increases the risk for chromosomal anomalies, cardiac defects, and the occurrence of twin-twin transfusion syndrome in monochorianic twins. Abnormal flow in the ductus venosus in about 80% of trisomy 21 fetuses and in about 5% of chromosomally normal fetuses [13].

6.4 Tricuspid Valve

Color and pulsed Doppler examination across the tricuspid valve is commonly used in the first trimester to assess for the presence of tricuspid valve regurgitation (TR). The presence of TR in the first trimester has been associated with chromosomal abnormalities [14, 15]. In the first trimester, TR is found in less than 5% of chromosomally normal fetuses, in more than 65% of fetuses with trisomy 21, and in more than 30% of fetuses with trisomy 18 [14]. Interrogation of other cardiac valves with color or pulsed Doppler is reserved for fetuses at risk for valve obstruction or when a cardiac malformation is suspected. Criteria for tricuspid valve evaluation at 11–13 + 6 weeks are- image should be such that the fetal thorax occupies most of the image (**Figure 4**). heart should be in apical position. Sample volume should be 2-3 mm should be positioned across the tricuspid valve with an angle should be less than 30 degrees from the direction of the interventricular septum. Significant TR is defined when regurgitation is more than half of the systole with velocity of >60 cm/s. The sweep speed should be 2-3 cm/s so that the wave forms are widely spread for better assessment. The tricuspid valve could be in sufficient in one or more of its three cusps, so, therefore the sample volume should be placed across the valve at least three times in an attempt to interrogate the complete valve [12].

6.5 Hepatic artery

It has been reported that high peak velocities in the hepatic artery are present in the first trimester in fetuses at risk for trisomy 21.

7. Second trimester soft markers

They are absent nasal bone, Aberrant subclavian artery, ventriculomegaly, increased Nuchal fold, Echogenic bowel loops, mild hydronephrosis, echogenic intra cardiac foci, short femur short humerus, choroid plexus cysts, single umbilical artery.

Major or minor abnormalities are found in about 75% of fetuses with trisomy 21 and in 10–15% of chromosomally normal fetuses. The Genetic sonogram is a targeted ultrasound looking for major abnormalities as well as minor markers for aneuploidy. Over the years these minor markers are being looked into and things like widened pelvic angle sandal gap deformity is going out of favour and is getting replaced by ARSA, pre nasal thickness and FMF angle. Absence of these markers decreases the risk of downs by around 70–80% but does not completely rule out Downs and hence Absence gives additional reassurance to the patient.

In first step when a soft marker is identified thoroughly search for other soft markers and structural abnormalities. In second step calculate the risk of aneuploidy based on likelihood ratios. This risk is calculated against background risk based maternal age alone or in combination with First trimester combined screening or second trimester quadruple test.

7.1 Increased nuchal fold

In second and third trimesters of pregnancy, abnormal accumulation of fluid behind the fetal neck can be known as nuchal cystic hygroma or nuchal edema. In about 75% of fetuses with cystic hygroma, there is a chromosomal abnormality and, in about 95% of cases, the abnormality is Turner syndrome. Chromosomal abnormalities are found in about one-third of the fetuses of nuchal edema and, in about 75% of cases, the abnormality is trisomy 21 or 18. Edema is also associated with fetal cardiovascular and pulmonary defects, skeletal dysplasia, congenital infections and metabolic and haematological disorders; The positive LR is 23.3 and negative LR is 0.8. Nuchal index is considered by some, because this is associated with gestational age. Nuchal index is (mean nuchal fold/mean BPD) x100 where the value of 11 or greater has a sensitivity of 50% and specificity of 96% (**Figure 6**).

7.2 Aberrant right subclavian artery (ARSA)

occurs in 0.5to 1.4%. four vessels arise from the aortic arch where the right subclavian artery arises from distal part of the aortic arch and courses behind the oesophagus and trachea to the right upper arm (**Figure 7**). ARSA is present in 1% of euploid fetuses and 24% of trisomy 21. ARSA is associated with other conotruncal

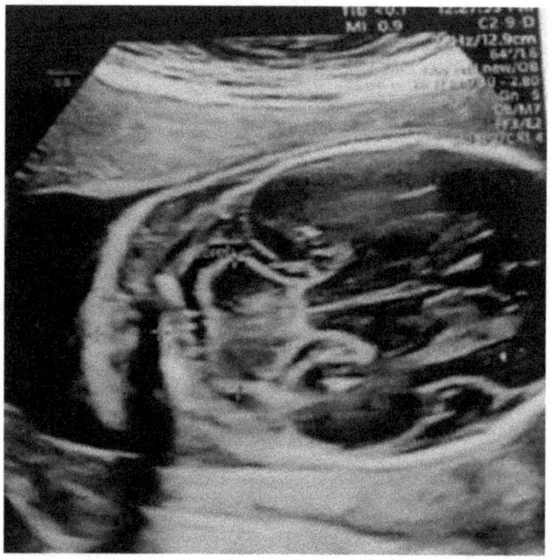

Figure 6.
Nuchal oedema.

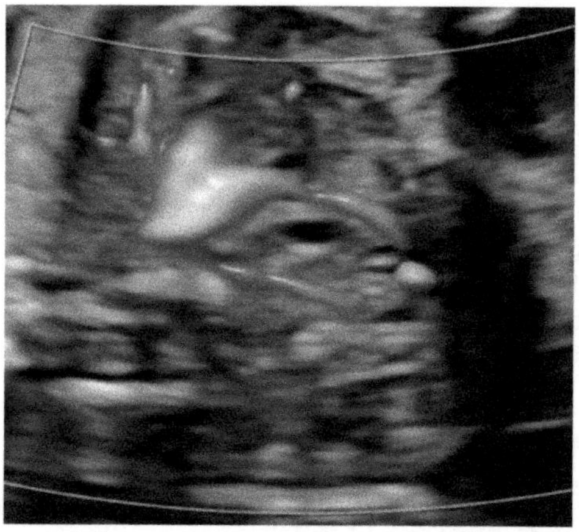

Figure 7.
ARSA.

anomalies increases the risk of microdeletion 22Q11 and other syndromes. The positive LR is 21.5 and negative LR is 0.71. when it is isolated LR is 3.9 times.

7.3 Echogenic bowel loop

This may be due to Swallowed blood, Cystic fibrosis or maternal infections. It may be also associated with congenital malformations of the bowel more so of upper GI lesions. And other perinatal complications, including fetal growth restriction. We have to also look for Ascites and bowel dilatation. Diagnosis of echogenic bowel should be confirmed by low frequency transducer, reduced Gain and without use of harmonics. Echogenicity should be equal to or more than bone (**Figure 8**). Grade 2 similar to bone echogenicity Grade 3 is more than bone. The positive LR of this is 11.4 and negative LR is 0.9.

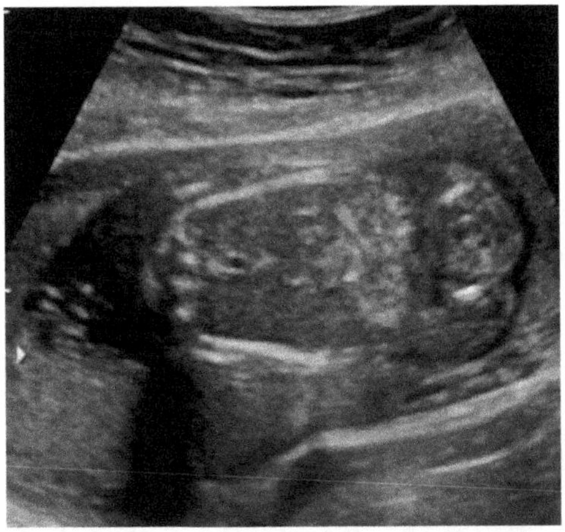

Figure 8.
Echogenic bowel loops.

7.4 Short femur/short Humerus

Short Femur and humerus is when the measurement is below 5th percentile for gestational age or measured/expected ratio < 0.9. The positive LR is 3.72 and negative LR is 0.8. regarding short humerus is the humerus measuring <2.5% or measured/expected ratio < 0.89. The Positive LR is 4.81 and negative LR is 0.74.

7.5 Echogenic intracardiac focus (EICF)

usually noted at region of papillary muscle 88% in Lt ventricle, 5%in rt. ventricle and 7% in biventricular. The echogenicity should be comparable to bone. Grading of EICF - Grade 2 similar echogenicity of bone and grade 3 more denser than bone (**Figure 9**). EICF in RV, biventricular, multiple and bright EICF are more associated

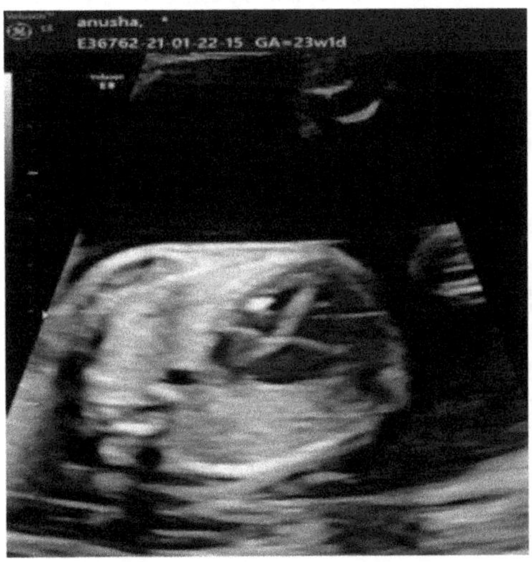

Figure 9.
EICF.

with aneuploidy, when compared to solitary LV EICF. The positive LR is 5.83 and negative LR is 0.8.

7.6 Mild ventriculomegaly

Normal ventricular measurements are <10 mm. If it is defined as mild ventriculomegaly when measurement is between 10 and 15 mm. (**Figure 10**). The overall prevalence of chromosomal defects in fetal ventriculomegaly is about 10% and the commonest chromosomal defects are trisomies 21, 18, 13 and triploidy. The positive LR is 27.52and negative LR is0.94.

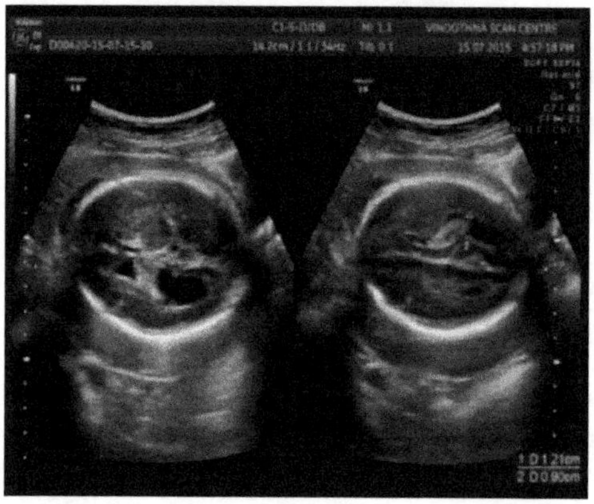

Figure 10.
Mild ventriculomegaly.

7.7 Mild hydronephrosis

pelvic AP diameter measuring >4 mm and it should be measured in transverse section in 12 clock or 6 clock position. The positive LR is 7.6 and negative LR is 0.92 (**Figure 11**).

There are other soft markers also those doesn't have any likely hood ratio but they are important and common in our practise but they are not a part of screening

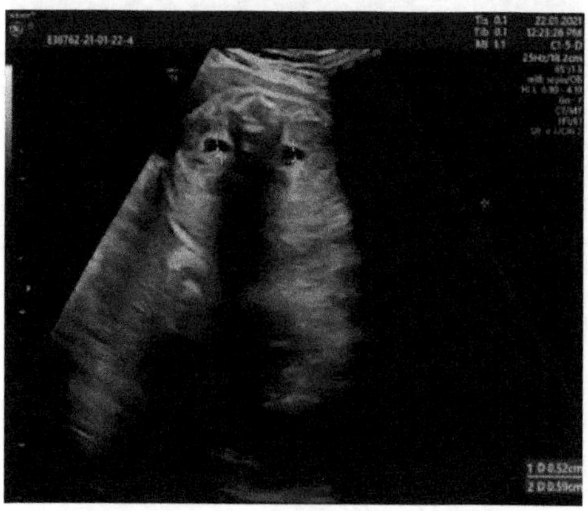

Figure 11.
Pyelectasis.

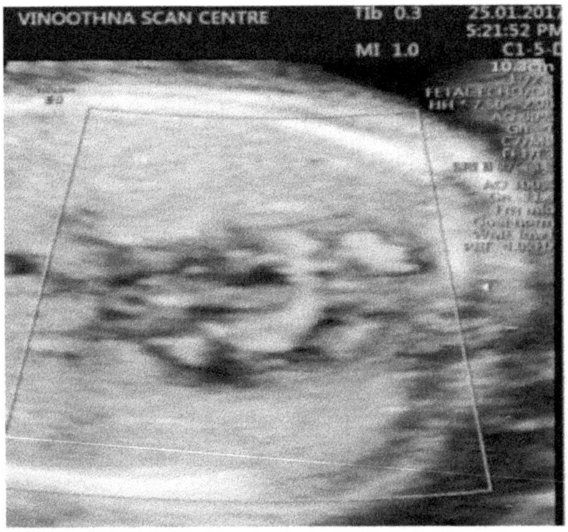

Figure 12.
Small membranous VSD.

protocol. They are the choroid plexus cysts and single umbilical artery, sandal gap toes, short ears, clinodactyly, increased iliac angle. Not only this Duodenal atresia and small membranous VSD (**Figure 12**) is also be associated with aneuploidy [16].

7.8 Choroid plexus cysts

they may be round or oval. May be unilateral or bilateral. They may be large or small. Commonly seen between 16 and 21 weeks by 23 week start undergoing regression. After 25–26 weeks uncommon to see. More commonly associated with trisomy 18. LR for trisomy 18 when isolated is 1.1–1.5.

7.9 Single umbilical artery

No strong association with aneuploidy. Usually associated with fetal cardiac, renal anomalies and oesophageal atresia (**Figure 13**).

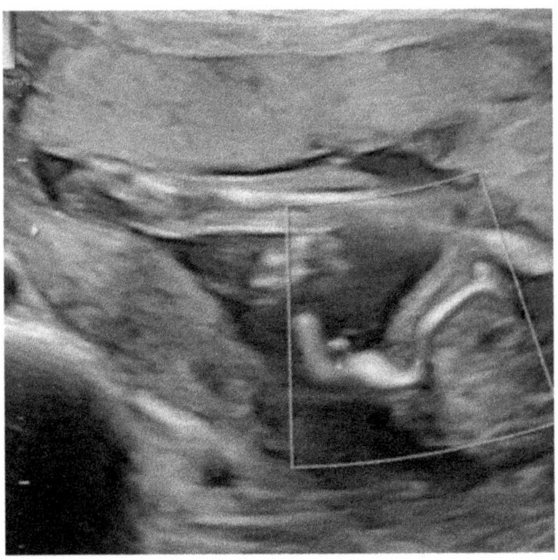

Figure 13.
Single umbilical artery.

7.10 Pre nasal thickness

In normal fetuses, the pre nasal thickness is small and the nasal bone is relatively long, resulting in a ratio of approximately 0.6 [17]. In trisomy 21 fetuses in the first trimester, the prenasal thickness increases, whereas the nasal bone length decreases, resulting in a ratio > 0.8 [17].

8. Non-invasive prenatal testing (NIPT)

Other names for NIPT are NIPS- non-invasive prenatal screening, cfDNA- cell free DNA. The test is based upon the presence of fetal cell-free DNA in the maternal circulation. Placental cell apoptosis releases into the maternal circulation as small DNA fragments (150-200 bp) that can be detected from >7 weeks of gestation [18]. It is estimated that about 2–20% of circulating cfDNA in the maternal circulation is fetal in origin [18]. So, about 1 in 10^3–10^7nucleated cells in maternal blood are fetal which can be enriched to about 1in 10–100 by techniques such as magnetic cell sorting (MACS) or fluorescence activated cell sorting (FACS) after attachment of magnetically labelled or fluorescent antibodies on to specific fetal cell surface markers. However, with the use of fluorescent *in situ* hybridization (FISH) and chromosome specific DNA probes it is possible to suspect fetal trisomy by the presence of three-signal nuclei in some of the cells of the maternal blood enriched for fetal cells. On the basis of currently available technology, examination of fetal cells from maternal blood is more likely to find an application as a method for assessment of risk. The sensitivity of NIPT is comparable to serum screening. Analysis of fetal cells from maternal blood is both labour intensive and requires highly skilled operators whereas in biochemical screening which is relatively easy to apply for mass population screening. The half-life of cfDNA is short and is typically undetectable within hours after delivery [19]. the detection rate for T21 is at 99% for a false-positive rate of 0.16% [20, 21]. Detection rate for T18 is at 97% for a false-positive rate of 0.15% [20]. The use of NIPT is rapidly expanding and is now being offered as the primary screening test in pregnancy. Even if the NIPT test has an excellent detection rate for T21, T18, and T13, other aneuploidies remain missed [22–24]. NIPT is a screening and not a diagnostic test so, caution should be used when NIPT is incorporated in the genetic evaluation of fetal malformations. Low fetal fraction is noted in High body mass and sampling before 10 weeks of gestation.in some laboratories fetal fraction <4% are considered too low to report a result which is often referred as a "no call "result. NIPT results depends on duration of gestation, number of fetuses and whether the fetus is live or not. For confirming number, gestational age and viability needs ultrasound examination before going for NIPT. If its low-risk population the positive predictive value of NIPT is low. False positive in NIPT are in placental mosaicism, vanishing Twin, maternal sex chromosome abnormality and Neoplasia. Even if NIPT is true positive it can-not distinguishes aneuploidy derived from translocation or disjunction type which is needed to know the recurrence risk for this again needs diagnostic test. Not only this the women who has no call report result needs comprehensive ultrasound evaluation and diagnostic tests because low fetal fraction may be associated with increased risk of aneuploidy.

9. Invasive fetal testing

1) **Chorionic villous sampling** should be done at 10–15 weeks. and overall fetal loss is 1%. This test can be done trans abdominal/trans vaginal approach and this

procedure should be done under ultrasound guidance and the sample is Trophoblast cells. Result comes within 48–72 hrs. Randomized studies have demonstrated that the rate of fetal loss following first-trimester transabdominal chorionic villus sampling is the same as with second-trimester amniocentesis. There is an association between chorionic villus sampling before 10 weeks to fetal transverse limb abnormalities, micrognathia and microglossia. It is therefore imperative that chorionic villus sampling is performed only after 11 weeks by appropriately trained operators.

2) **Amniocentesis** should be done at 15–20 weeks. In this we introduce needle inside the amniotic cavity to extract the amniotic fluid. Sampling cells are amniocytes, fetal dermal fibroblasts. Karyotype results take 7–10 days, and overall fetal loss is 0.5%.

3) **cordocentesis** (per cutaneous umbilical blood sampling) which should be done at >18-20 weeks. Under ultrasound guidance needle should be introduced into the cord near the placental insertion. Sampling should be done from umbilical vein. Sampling cells are fetal blood cells sampled from umbilical vein and overall fetal loss is 1.5–3%. In a randomized study, 4,606 low-risk, healthy women, 25–34 years old, at 14–20 weeks of gestation, were randomly allocated to amniocentesis or ultrasound examination alone [25]. The total fetal loss rate in the patients having amniocentesis was 1% higher than in the controls. The study also reported that amniocentesis was associated with an increased risk of respiratory distress syndrome and pneumonia. Randomized studies have demonstrated that after early amniocentesis i.e., around 10–14 weeks of gestation the rate of fetal loss is about 2% higher and the incidence of talipes equinovarus is 1.6% higher than the first-trimester chorionic villus sampling or second-trimester amniocentesis. It was apparent that amniocentesis carried a risk of miscarriage and this in conjunction with the financial cost implications, meant that prenatal diagnosis could not be offered to the entire pregnant population.

10. Sonographic and biochemical features of Aneuploidy

10.1 Trisomy 21

Factors that is associated with an increased risk of "Down syndrome" are higher maternal age, a parental translocation involving chromosome 21, previous child with T21, significant ultrasound findings and a positive screening test result. In pregnancies with T21 fetuses, the maternal serum concentration of free β-HCG is about twice (about 2MoM) as high and PAPP-A is reduced to half (about 0.5 MoM) compared to euploid pregnancies. Although NT measurement alone identifies about 75–80% of T21 fetuses, the combination of NT with maternal biomarkers in the first trimester increases the T21 detection rate to 85–95%, while keeping the false-positive rate at 5%. AFP is decreased in T21.

In addition to NT, other sensitive first trimester ultrasound markers of T21 include absence or hypoplasia of the nasal bone (60–70%), increased impedance to flow in the ductus venosus (about 80%), tricuspid regurgitation, cardiac malformations (atrioventricular septal defect) with or without generalized edema, aberrant right subclavian artery and echogenic intracardiac focus. Increased fronto maxillary fascial angle (short maxilla in 25%), renal pylectasis and echogenic bowel loops are also soft markers for "Down syndrome" (**Table 3**) (**Figures 14–18**).

In second trimester scan the soft markers in Trisomy 21 are nasal hypoplasia, increased nuchal fold thickness, intracardiac echogenic foci, echogenic bowel, hydronephrosis, shortening of the femur and more so of the humerus. It may also be

	Trisomy21	Trisomy18	Trisomy13	Triploidy	Turner
Ventriculomegaly	+	+	+	+	
Holoprocencephaly			+		
Choroid plexus cyst		+			
Dandy walker complex		+	+		
Fascial cleft		+	+		
micrognathia		+		+	
Nasal hypoplasia	+				
Nuchal edema	+	+	+		
Cystic hygroma					+
Diaphragmatic hernia		+	+		
Cardiac defect	+	+	+	+	+
Exomphalos		+	+		
Duodenal atresia	+				
Esophageal atresia	+	+			
Renal defects	+	+	+	+	+
Short limbs	+	+		+	+
Clinodactyly	+				
Overlapping fingers		+			
polydactyly			+		
syndactyly				+	
Talipes		+	+	+	
Fetal growth restriction		+		+	+

Source: Snijders and Nicolaides 1996, Nicolaides et al. 1992.

Table 3.
Common chromosomal defects in fetuses with sonographic abnormalities [9, 26].

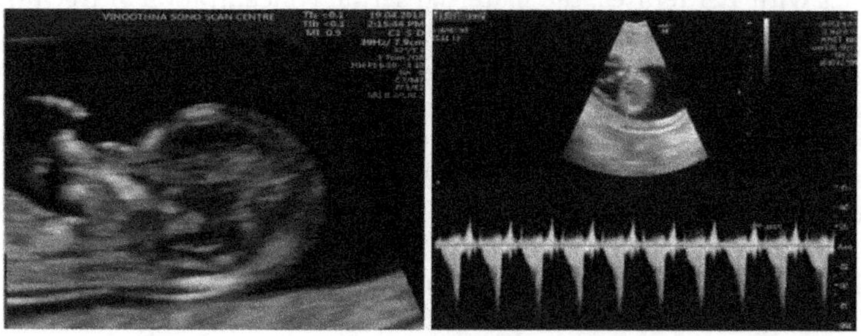

Figure 14.
T21 Fetus of 12 weeks 3 days showing normal NT with AFNB and Tricuspid regurgitation.

associate with cardiac defects, duodenal atresia, sandal gap and clinodactyly or mid-phalanx hypoplasia of the fifth finger. Trisomy 21 is found in about 40% of cases of duodenal atresia.

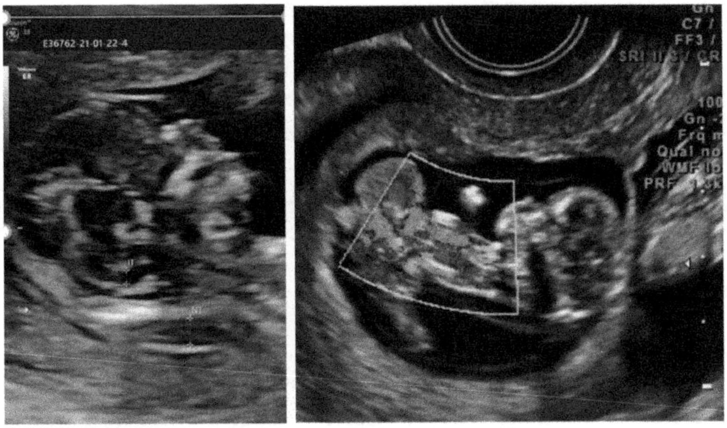

Figure 15.
T21 fetus of 13 weeks 5 days showing increased NT with Omphalocele.

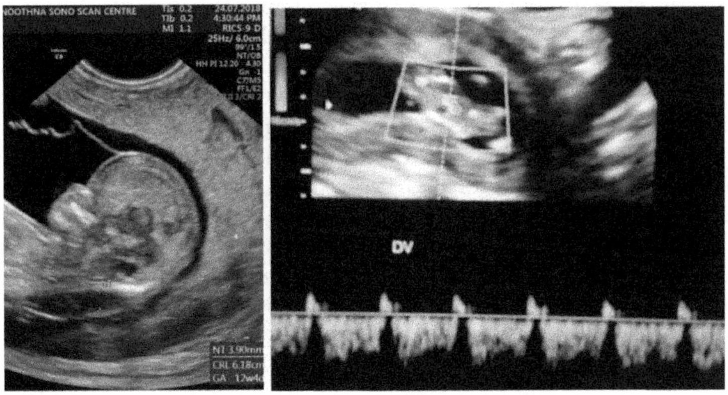

Figure 16.
T21 fetus showing Increased NT with dilated posterior fossa and reverse flow in ductus venosus.

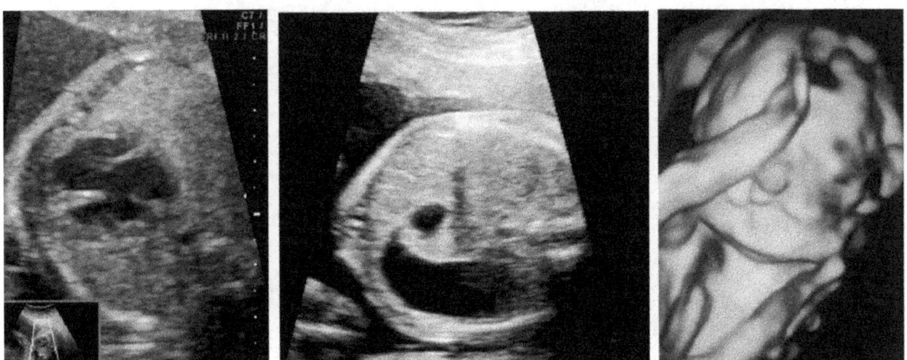

Figure 17.
T21 with Atrioventricular septal defect with duodenal atresia(double bubble sign) and cleft lip with palate.

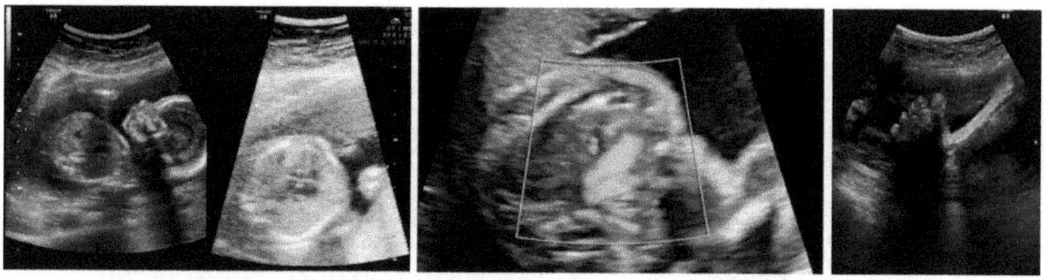

Figure 18.
T21 with Absent nasal bone with EIC, ARSA and club foot.

10.2 Trisomy 18 and Trisomy13

Thickened NT is a common first trimester findings in Aneuploidy. In T18 and T13, NT median values were shown to be 5.5 and 4.0 mm, respectively [16, 27]. Reduced PAPP-A value in both trisomies noted with a median value of 0.2 MoM for T18 and 0.3 MoM for T13. Free β-HCG values are decreased whereas it is increased in T21. In T18 and T13 median values of free β-HCG 0.2 MoM and 0.5 MoM, respectively. T18 or T13 is often first suspected by the presence of typical ultrasound features, rather than by biochemical screening (**Figures 19–25**). single umbilical artery is found 80% fetuses with T18 and in about 3% of chromosomally normal fetuses [28]. There is 7fold increased risk of T18 associated with single umbilical artery noted. Presence of megacystis After taking into account maternal age and fetal NT the increases the likelihood for trisomy 13 or 18 by a factor of 6.7.

Presence of exomphalos in association with T18 in first trimester is 60% compared about 30% at mid gestation and 15% in neonates. Trisomy 13 and Turner syndrome are associated with tachycardia, whereas in trisomy 18 and triploidy there is fetal bradycardia [29]. pulsatile flow in the umbilical vein is noted in 90% of fetuses in T18 and T13 where as 25% of chromosomally normal fetuses. The prevalence of chromosomal defects in Dandy walker -complex is about 40%, mainly in trisomies 18, 13 and triploidy.

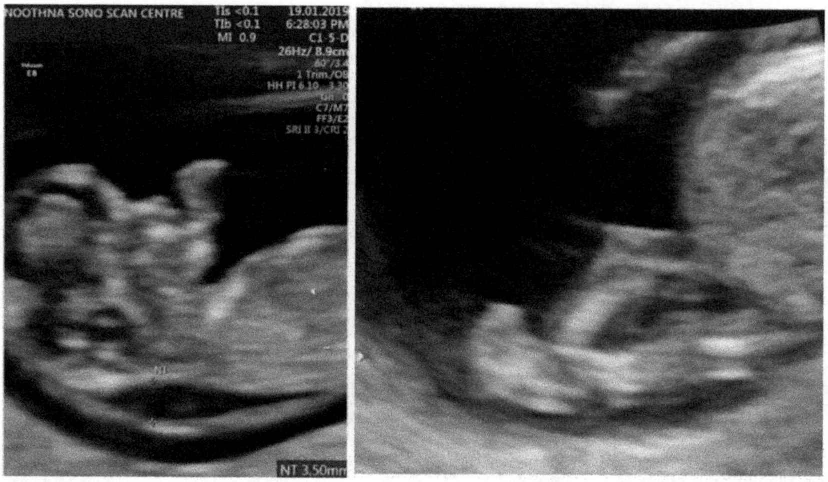

Figure 19.
T18 12 weeks 1 day showing increased NT, absent nasal bone, cleft lip and palate and Congenital talipes equinovarus.

DOI: http://dx.doi.org/10.5772/intechopen.96757

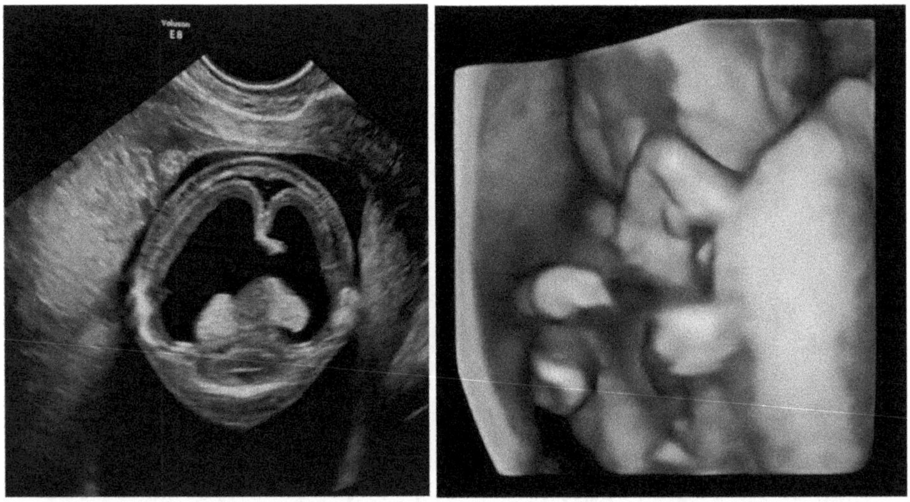

Figure 20.
T18 fetus of 15 weeks gestational age with Holoprocencephaly and radial ray abnormality.

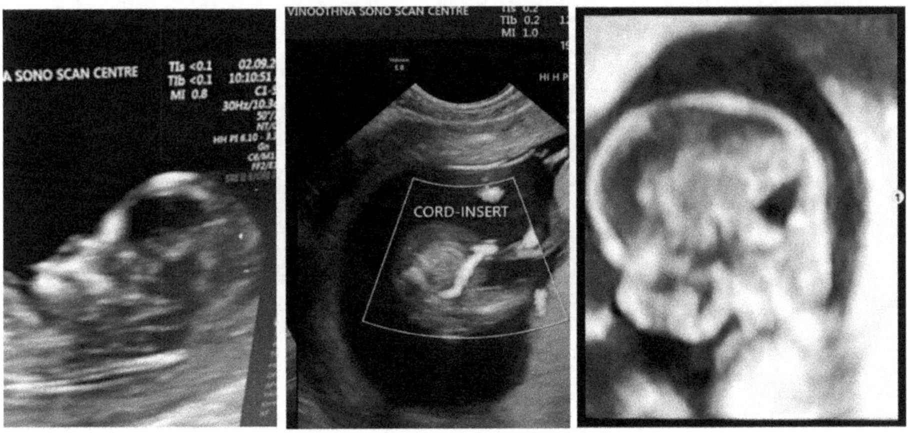

Figure 21.
T18 fetus showing normal NT with dilated posterior fossa and single umbilical artery at 13 weeks 2 days followup 3D at 16 weeks 4 days with vermian rotation and incread Brainstem vermian angle.

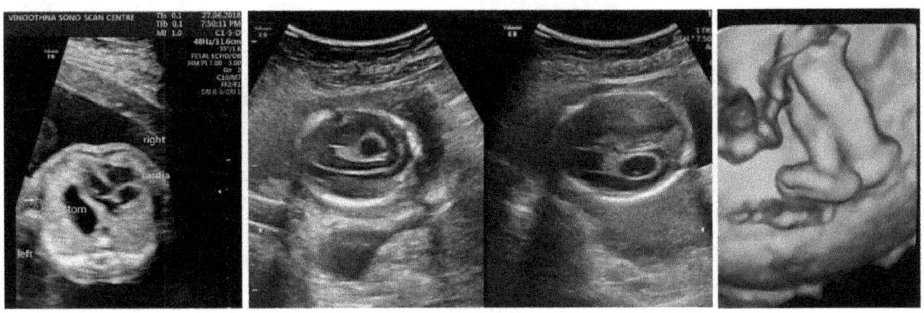

Figure 22.
Fetus of T18 showing Diaphragmatic hernia, choroid plexus cysts and bilateral rocker bottom foot at 21 weeks 5 days gestation.

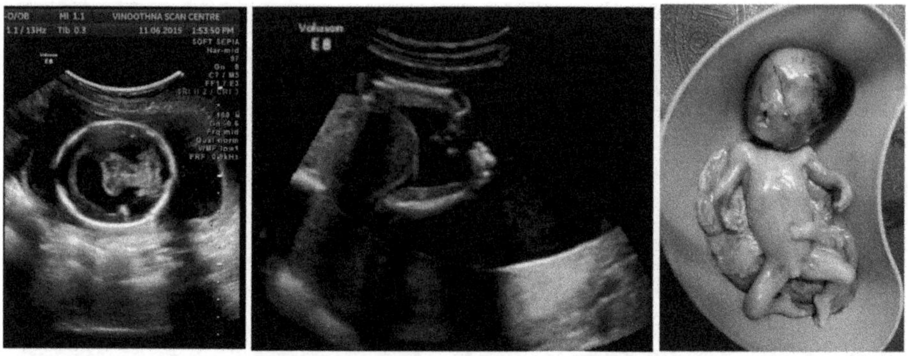

Figure 23.
15 weeks 5 days fetus of T13 showing holoprocencephaly, club hands and aborted fetus showing midline cleft with proboscis anophthalmia and bilateral club hands.

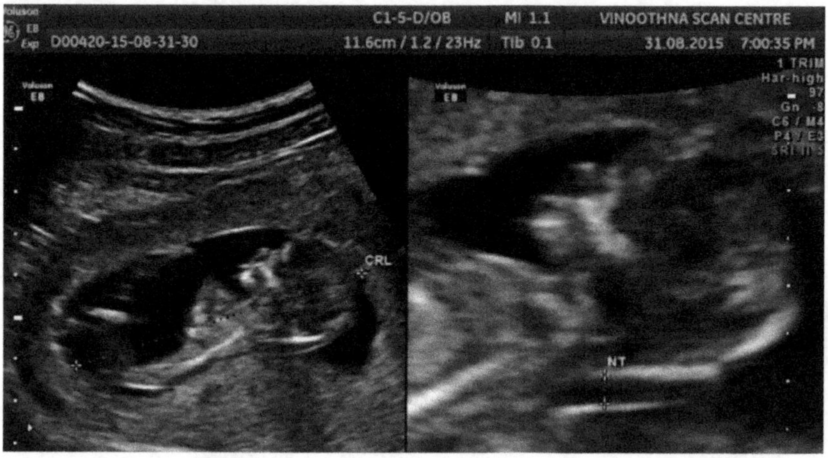

Figure 24.
Megacystits with increased NT of 12 weeks 1 day T13 fetus.

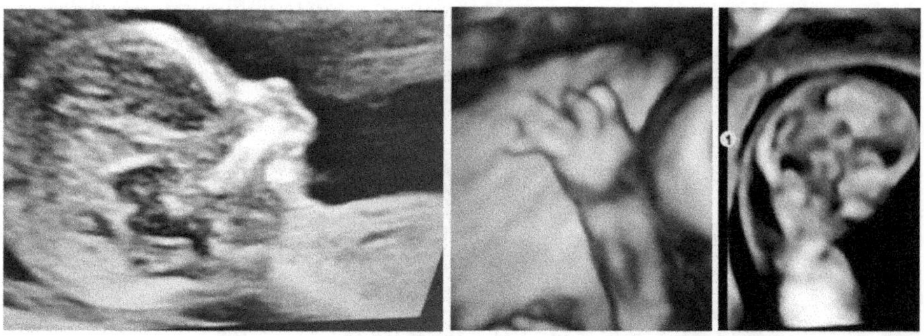

Figure 25.
15 weeks 3 days fetus showing micrognathia with polydactyly and syndactyly. In another fetus of 14 weeks 2 days 3D showing increased NT with posterior fossa dilatation and micrognathia in T13 cases.

20% 0f diaphragmatic hernia is associated with chromosomal defects mainly withTrisomy18. Heart abnormalities are found in more than 90% of fetuses with trisomy 18 or 13 and 40% of those with trisomy 21 or Turner syndrome. 30% and 15%

cases of Exomphalos at mid gestation and in neonates are associated with Chromosomal defects, mainly trisomies 18 and 13. The prevalence of chromosomal defects is four-times higher when the exomphalos sac contains only bowel than in cases where the liver is included. Prenatally 20% of oesophageal atresia cases are associated with chromosomal defects, mainly trisomy 18. Polydactyly is associated with trisomy 13, overlapping fingers, Talipes and rocker bottom feet are associated with trisomy 18. Usually, Trisomy 18 and triploidy are associated with moderately severe growth restriction whereas trisomy 13, Turner syndrome with mild growth restriction and in trisomy 21 growth is essentially normal [30]. In second trimester scan Trisomy 18 is associated with strawberry-shaped head, choroid plexus cysts, absent corpus callosum, enlarged cisterna magna, facial cleft, micrognathia, nuchal edema, heart defects, esophageal atresia, diaphragmatic hernia and usually exomphalos with bowel only in the sac. The other associated findings are single umbilical artery, renal abnormalities, echogenic bowel, myelomeningocele, growth restriction and shortening of the limbs, radial aplasia, overlapping fingers and talipes or rocker bottom feet.

Trisomy 13 is associated with microcephaly, holoprosencephaly, facial abnormalities, cardiac abnormalities, exomphalos, enlarged and echogenic kidneys and post axial polydactyly.

11. Monosomy X (turner syndrome)

NT has a median value of 7.8 mm [16] and has often been described as a cystic hygroma (**Figure 26**). The occurrence of monosomy X is not related to maternal age. Typically, lymphatic disturbances in turner syndrome are not limited to the neck region but involve the whole body including the presence of skin edema, hydrothorax and ascites. Generally Normal Nasal bone is present in fetuses with monosomy X [31]. Normal maternal serum-free β-HCG (1.1 MoM) and low PAPP-A is noted (0.49 MoM) [32]. Typical sonographic features in monosomy X includes large nuchal cystic hygromas, generalised edema, mild pleural effusions and ascites, cardiac abnormalities like left ventricular outflow tract obstruction, fetal tachycardia and renal anomalies such as the presence of horseshoe kidneys.

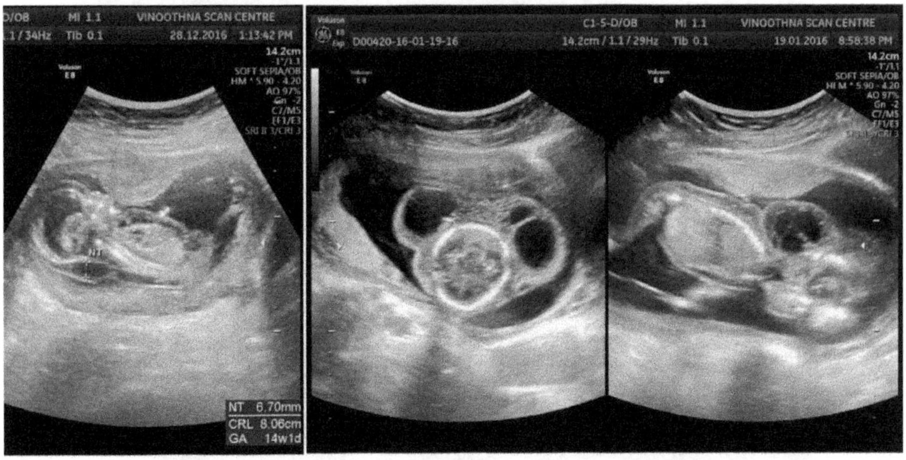

Figure 26.
2 different cases of turners syndrome with generalised edema and cystic hygroma.

11.1 Triploidy

In triploidy, there is a complete additional haploid set of chromosomes resulting in 69 chromosomes in each cell instead of 46 chromosomes. The additional haploid set can be of paternal or maternal origin. The “paternal” type is called diandric triploidy and the “maternal” type is called digynic triploidy. These two types show different features, which can be often differentiated on ultrasound. The typical pattern of diandric triploidy includes the presence of a normally grown fetus with molar placenta, whereas in digynic triploidy, severe growth restriction is noted with a small but not molar placenta. Profile of biochemistry is different in both types due to these placental differences. Diandric triploidy is associated with increased maternal serum-free β-HCG and mildly decreased PAPP-A and in digynic triploidy which is associated with markedly decreased maternal serum free β-HCG and PAPP-A. Significantly short CRL with marked difference in size between the abdominal and head circumference, typically of more than 2 weeks of gestational age [33] which is a pathognomonic sign of digynic triploidy (**Figure 27**). In second trimester scan Triploidy where the extra set of chromosomes is paternally derived is associated with a molar placenta and the pregnancy rarely persists beyond 20 weeks. When there is a double maternal chromosome contribution, the pregnancy may persist into the third trimester (**Figure 27**). Commonly there is mild

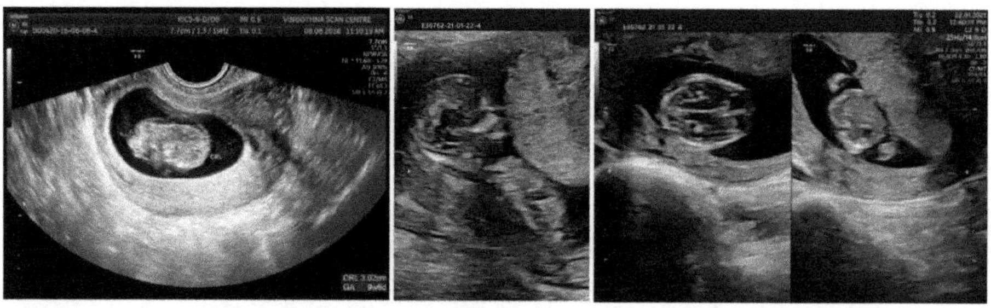

Figure 27.
Two fetuses of Digynic Triploidy showing short CRL with size difference in abdominal head circumference.

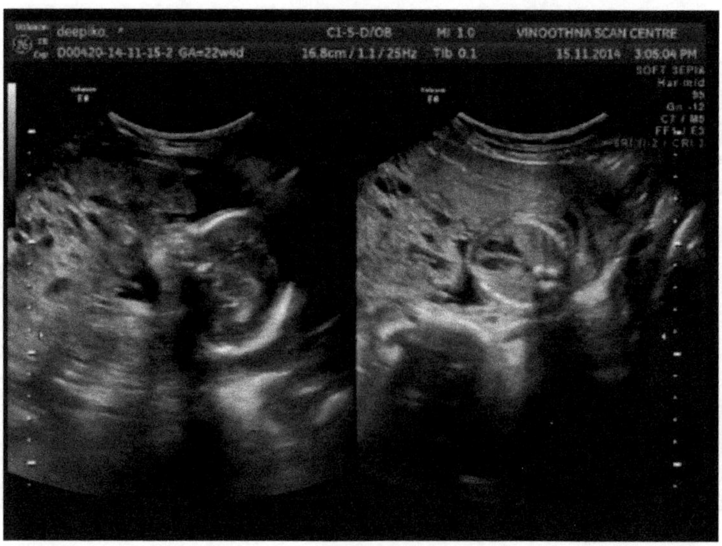

Figure 28.
Live fetus at 22 weeks 4 days with Molar changes in placenta in a diandric triploidy.

ventriculomegaly, micrognathia, cardiac abnormalities, myelomeningocele, syndactyly, and 'hitch-hiker' toe deformity (**Figure 28**).

12. Risk assessment in first and second trimester

The risk for trisomies in women who have had a previous fetus or child with a trisomy is higher than the one expected on the basis of their age alone.

when we have only CRL, NT, maternal age without biochemical markers there are calculators where we can enter these measurements, we get the risk assessment for downs at the time of birth- Pregnancy calculators- EDD. We can do same thing with only 2nd trimester markers without biochemical or first trimester screen results for this we will take the LR+ value of each marker present and LR- values of all absent markers and multiple all of these to get the LR for combination [8].

Instead if we find any soft markers we enter the same into the excel sheet provided by [8] M. Agathokleous et al. Excel sheet for downs.

Meta- analysis of second-trimester markers for trisomy21 [8] M. Agathokleous et al., ultrasound obstet Gynecol 2013;41:247–261.

For example:-.

when we get the measurements, we apply the same into the calculators and get the risk assessment for downs at the time of birth. It is given as in 1 in ————.

>1in 19(high risk): offer invasive testing.

>1in 50(high risk): offer NIPT/Invasive testing.

<1in 1000(Low risk): Back to routine second trimester genetic sonogram.

1in 50-1in 999(intermediate risk): Assess NB, DV, TR and recalculate risk+/-NIPT.

New cut-of risk for downs as 1:250, borderline between 251 and 1000, and less risk if <1:1001.

First trimester between 11 and 13 weeks 6 days scan evaluate NT, nasal bone along with Tricuspid valve regurgitation, a wave in Ductus Venosus and other major structural defects. Not only this detail cardiac evaluation should be done. If there is no abnormality repeat scan at 18–22 weeks may be recommended. In the second trimester scan look for soft markers, if there is any marker or abnormality detailed anatomy scan and echocardiography. In case of most isolated markers including intra cardiac echogenic focus, echogenic Bowel, mild hydronephrosis and short femur, there is only a small effect on modifying the pre-test odds.

All these are only screening protocols they are not diagnostic so, fetal karyotyping option is aways open to either risk groups.

Previous affected Pregnancy.

In women who had a previous pregnancy with trisomy 21, the risk of recurrence in the subsequent pregnancy is 0.75% higher than the maternal and gestational age-related risk for trisomy 21 at the time of testing. Recurrence is chromosome specific. If a previous pregnancy is T21 the result will be classified as screen positive regardless of level of screening markers. Risk is calculated which takes account of a women's age at the time of her previous pregnancy with "Down syndrome" for the risk calculation.

"Down syndrome" may be non-disjunction type (95%) where there is a recurrence rate of 1% where as in translocation type like (21–21) if either parent is carrying same type of translocation then there is 100% rate of recurrence.

If there is h/o prior affected downs child screening test is not reassuring her so, better to go for direct invasive testing if she comes at first trimester go for CVS.

In Twin gestation.

Dichorionic twin- Free β-HCG and PAPP-A levels are nearly twice as high as singleton. Calculate the risk for each fetus based on maternal age and fetal NT. If one fetus the NT is increased look for other markers. Detection rate is 75–80%.

In monozygotic twins' risk is same as singleton pregnancies.

In monochorionic twin pregnancies raised NT is an early manifestation of TTTS. So, false positive rate will be increased. Free beta HCG and PAPP-A levels are lower than dichorionic twin to twin transfusion syndrome as well as for chromosomal abnormality.

Calculate the risk of each fetus based on NT, serum biochemistry and then the average risk between the two fetuses is considered as whole.

No method is accurate for screening of fetal aneuploidy as it is in singleton pregnancy.

Appropriate Models for aneuploidy detection:

- Age (not recommended).
- CRL & NIPT (Ideal for first trimester, misses advantages of first trimester scan and expensive)
- Age, CRL & NT (skill)
- Age & Biochemistry (poor detection rate)
- Age + CRL + Maternal factors +NT + PAPP-A + HCG (combined test)
- Age + Maternal factors + CRL + NT + Additional markers + Biochemistry (enhanced sensitivity and low FPR but need time and skill)
- First trimester combined test + second trimester Quad (sequential or integrated)
- First trimester Quad: Age + historical factors + PAPP-A + βHCG + PIGF +AFP (risk for pre-eclampsia and NTD)
- First trimester Penta: Combined test + Nasal bone + AFP + DIA + PIGF (high detection rate and low FPR).

13. Conclusion

In the economically privileged patient first trimester screening should include an 11–14 weeks complete assessment with first trimester combined screen, PIGF and NIPT. For population screening is by combined screening. Woman with positive screen test result should be counselled and offered the option of diagnostic testing. Those who have a negative test results should be counselled regarding their lower adjusted risk. Even if a woman has low risk results, she may choose diagnostic testing later in pregnancy whenever there is fetal anomalies or markers on follow-up sonography.

Acknowledgements

The authors wish to express thanks to all parentages involved for giving permission to collect the presented data. The authors also wish to express their thanks to Dr. Ashok Khurana, Dr. TLN Praveen and Dr. Krishna Gopal for the source of information.

Author details

Madhavilatha Routhu[1*] and Shiva Surya Varalakshmi Koneru[2]

1 Kakatiya Medical College, Warangal, India

2 Shiva Hospital, Warangal, India

*Address all correspondence to: madhaviradiologist@gmail.com

References

[1] Benacerraf BR, Frigoletto FD. Soft tissue nuchal fold in the second-trimester fetus: standards for normal measurements compared with those in "Down syndrome". Am J Obstet Gynecol. 1987;157:1146–1149. [PubMed] [Google Scholar]

[2] Nicolaides KH, Azar G, Byrne D, Mansur C, Marks K. Fetal nuchal translucency: ultrasound screening for chromosomal defects in first trimester of pregnancy. BMJ 1992;304:867–869.

[3] Bindra R, Heath V, Liao A, Spencer K, Nicolaides KH. One stop clinic for assessment of risk for trisomy 21 at 11–14 weeks: A prospective study of 15,030 pregnancies. Ultrasound Obstet Gynecol 2002;20:219–225.

[4] Spencer K, Spencer CE, Power M, Dawson C, Nicolaides KH. Screening for chromosomal abnormalities in the first trimester using ultrasound and maternal serum biochemistry in a one stop clinic: A review of three years prospective experience. BJOG 2003b;110:281–286.

[5] Cuckle HS, Malone FD, Wright D, Porter TF, Nyberg DA, Comstock CH, et al. Contingent screening for "Down syndrome"—results from the Faster trial. Prenat Diagn 2008;28:89-94.(Level II-3).

[6] Baer RJ, Flessel MC, Jelliffe-Pawlowski LL, Goldman S,Hudgins L, Hull AD, et al. Detection rates for aneuploidy by first-trimester and sequential screening. Obstet Gynecol 2015;126:753-9. (Level II-3).

[7] https://journals.lww.com/greenjournal/Fulltext/2016/05000/PracticeBulletinNo163ScreeningforFetal.41.aspx.

[8] Meta- analysis of second-trimester markers for trisomy21 M.Agathokleous et al, ultrasound obstet Gynecol 2013;41: 247-261.

[9] Snijders RJM, Nicolaides KH. Sequential screening. In: Nicolaides KH, editor. Ultrasound markers for fetal chromosomal defects. Carnforth, UK: Parthenon Publishing, 1996, pp109–13.

[10] Chasen ST, Skupski DW, McCullough LB, Chervenak FA. Prenatal informed consent for sonogram: the time for first-trimester nuchal translucency has come. J Ultrasound Med 2001;20:1147–1152.

[11] Snijders RJM, Noble P, Sebire N, Souka A, Nicolaides KH. UK multicentre project on assessment of risk of trisomy 21 by maternal age and fetal nuchal translucency thickness at 10–14 weeks of gestation. Lancet 1998;351:343–346.

[12] Nicolaides KH. The fetal medicine foundation. Available from: https://fetalmedicine.org. Accessed March 1, 2017.

[13] Nicolaides KH. Nuchal translucency and other first-trimester sonographic markers of chromosomal abnormalities. Am J Obstet Gynecol 2004;191:45–67.

[14] Falcon O, Faiola S, Huggon I, et al. Fetal tricuspid regurgitation at the 11 + 0 to 13 + 6-week scan: association with chromosomal defects and reproducibility of the method. Ultrasound Obstet Gynecol. 2006;27:609–612.

[15] Khalil A, Nicolaides KH. Fetal heart defects: potential and pitfalls of first-trimester detection. Semin Fetal Neonatal Med. 2013;18:251–260.

[16] Nicolaides KH. Screening for fetal aneuploidies at 11 to 13 weeks. Prenat Diagn.2011;31:7–15.

[17] Manegold-Brauer G, Bourdil L, Berg C, et al. Prenasal thickness to nasal bone length ratio in normal and trisomy 21 fetuses at 11-14 weeks of gestation. Prenat Diagn. 2015;35:1079–1084.

[18] Illanes S, Denbow M, Kailasam C, et al. Early detection of cell-free fetal DNA in maternal plasma. Early Hum Dev. 2007;83:563–566.

[19] Lo YM, Zhang J, Leung TN, et al. Rapid clearance of fetal DNA from maternal plasma. Am J Hum Genet. 1999;64:218–224.

[20] Lo JO, Cori DF, Norton ME, et al. Noninvasive prenatal testing. Obstet Gynecol Surv. 2014;69:89–99.

[21] Norton ME, Jacobsson B, Swamy GK, et al. Cell-free DNA analysis for noninvasive examination of trisomy. N Engl J Med. 2015;372:1589–1597.

[22] Syngelaki A, Pergament E, Homfray T, et al. Replacing the combined test by cellfree DNA testing in screening for trisomies 21, 18 and 13: impact on the diagnosis of other chromosomal abnormalities. Fetal Diagn Ther. 2014;35:174–184.

[23] Norton ME, Baer RJ, Wapner RJ, et al. Cell-free DNA vs sequential screening for the detection of fetal chromosomal abnormalities. Am J Obstet Gynecol.2016;214:727.e1–.e6.

[24] Wellesley D, Dolk H, Boyd PA, et al. Rare chromosome abnormalities, prevalence and prenatal diagnosis rates from population-based congenital anomaly registers in Europe. Eur J Hum Genet. 2012;20:521–526.

[25] Tabor A, Philip J, Madsen M, Bang J, Obel EB, Norgaard-Pedersen B. Randomised controlled trial of genetic amniocentesis in 4,606 low-risk women. Lancet 1986;1:1287–1293.

[26] Nicolaides KH, Snijders RJM, Gosden RJM, Berry C, Campbell S. Ultrasonographically detectable markers of fetal chromosomal abnormalities. Lancet 1992;340:704–707.

[27] Santorum M, Wright D, Syngelaki A, et al. Accuracy of first trimester combined test in screening for trisomies 21, 18 and 13. Ultrasound Obstet Gynecol. 2016.doi:10.1002/uog.17283.

[28] Rembouskos G, Cicero S, Longo D, Sacchini C, Nicolaides KH. Single Umbilical Artery at 11–14 weeks: relation to chromosomal defects. Ultrasound Obstet Gynecol 2003;22: 567–570.

[29] Liao AW, Snijders R, Geerts L, Spencer K, Nicolaides KH. Fetal heart rate in chromosomally abnormal fetuses. Ultrasound Obstet Gynecol 2000;16:610–613.

[30] Nicolaides KH, Sebire NJ, Snijders JM. Crown rump length in chromosomally abnormal fetuses. In Nicolaides KH (Ed) The 11–14-week scan-The diagnosis of fetal abnormalities. New York: Parthenon Publishing, 1996, pp31–3.

[31] Wagner P, Sonek J, Hoopmann M, et al. First-trimester screening for trisomies 18 and 13, triploidy and Turner syndrome by detailed early anomaly scan. Ultrasound Obstet Gynecol. 2016;48:446–451.

[32] Spencer K, Tul N, Nicolaides KH. Maternal serum free beta-hCG and PAPP-A in fetal sex chromosome defects in the first trimester. Prenat Diagn. 2000;20:390–394.

[33] Zalel Y, Shapiro I, Weissmann-Brenner A, et al. Prenatal sonographic features of triploidy at 12–16 weeks. Prenat Diagn. 2016;36:650–655.

Chapter 10

Background, Diagnosis, Types, Management/Prevention and Implications of Chromosomal Abnormalities

Subhadra Poornima, Saranya Vadrevu and Imran Ali Khan

Abstract

Chromosomal abnormalities are caused by both meiotic and mitotic errors, and can be found in both reproductive and somatic cells. Meiotic and mitotic errors, on the other hand, may result in the development of abnormal copies of chromosomes. Somatic cell chromosomal abnormalities cause mosaicism, which implies that certain cells are normal while others express the abnormality. Fascinating genetic chromosomal discoveries have given answers to mysteries in children suffering from premature growth/retardation, ambiguous genitalia, metabolic disorders, dysmorphic syndromes, primary amenorrhea, infertility, recurrent pregnancy loss, and cancers. Many factors influence the risk of chromosomal abnormalities, including advanced maternal age, environmental factors such as smoking, alcohol intake, and exposure to chemicals/radiation, and family history. It is an inevitable fact that majority of chromosomal abnormalities arise spontaneously and are not treatable. Much attention has not been devoted to the study of chromosomal abnormalities in order to better understand the pathogenesis and rising prevalence of various clinical conditions. This chapter will address the relationship of chromosomal abnormalities in various conditions with the goal of increasing awareness of causes and furthering diagnosis, management/treatment, counseling, and prevention options. Furthermore, preimplantation and prenatal testing can be planned from the laboratory bench to the clinical bedside using sophisticated molecular techniques.

Keywords: Chromosomal abnormalities, Counseling, management, Prenatal, Infertility

1. Introduction

Genetic material exists as a compact mass in relatively confined volume at cellular level as chromatin within the nucleus and the packaging of the chromatin is flexible and changes during the cell cycle. At the time of division, interphase chromatin becomes firmly packed, and individual chromosomes become visible as separate entities. A chromosome is a component for segregating genetic material during the cell division process. A structure known as a centromere is observed in the chromosome [1]. Kinetochore is a structure that connects the centromere to microtubules at the broader cellular level. A eukaryotic chromosome is made up of long linear segments of DNA, as well as telomeres, which anchor the ends and are stretched by a specific mechanism that avoids the challenges of replicating the ends of linear DNA.

Chromatin has a scattered appearance, i.e. euchromatin, and includes the bulk of transcriptionally active genes. Some chromatin sections are densely packed, which is known as heterochromatin, and are normally inactive transcriptionally. The building blocks of chromatin are nucleosomes, which comprise 200 base pairs of DNAs arranged by an octamer in the basic proteins in a bead-like shape. Histones are protein components that form an inner core (**Figure 1**). The coiling of nucleosomes into a helical form present in interphase chromatin as well as mitotic chromosomes is the second level of organization [2]. Euchromatin is cyclically interchangeable with mitotic chromosomal packing, which is much more compact. Heterochromatin is equally dense in the packing of mitotic chromosomes. The chromatin mass includes up to double the protein content of DNA. Changes in chromatin structure are achieved through interaction with new proteins or through alterations to existing chromosomal proteins. Non-histone proteins include chromatin proteins other than histones that are transferable between tissues and species.

Each chromosome has a single long helix of DNA that is folded into a fiber and runs the length of the chromosome. Various chromosomes have different banding patterns; certain staining procedures allow chromosomes to look as a sequence of striations known as G bands. Bands typically have lower GC content than interbands, and genes are clustered in the GC rich region. Each chromosome's distinctive banded structure is caused by the folding of deoxy ribonucleoprotein fiber. The microtubules attached to the kinetochores forming in its central section's hold chromosome on the mitotic spindle. Centromeres contain heterochromatin, which is densely packed with satellite DNA sequences. A centromere is essential for segregation, and a single break produces one piece with the centromere and an acrocentric fragment. A telomere is crucial for chromosomal end stability. It is made up of simple repeats in which a C + A rich strand has the sequence C (A/T). The telomere is reproduced by a particular process, usually the complement of template RNA primers in the telomere, which generates a primer that is expanded by enzyme reverse transcriptase activity [3].

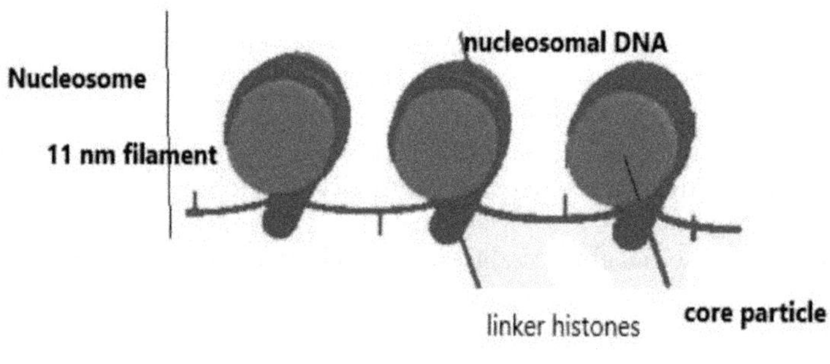

Figure 1.
Chromatin structure, nucleosome, and histone proteins are depicted in a cartoon.

1.1 Chromosome

Chromosomes are thread-like structures packed with histone proteins that contain the genetic material from which children inherit features from their parents. Deoxyribose nucleic acid (DNA) generates proteins that aid in human growth and development. Humans have 23 pairs of chromosomes, which are separated into autosomes (22 pairs) and allosomes (one pair as X and Y). Chromosomes divide to generate gametes during meiotic division. Homologous chromosomes are a set of chromosomes (23 pairs = 46 chromosomes) inherited from the maternal side and the other from the paternal side [4].

1.2 Types of chromosomes

Each chromosome possesses a centromere, which is critical for chromosome placement and visible during metaphase. The centromere separates the chromosomes into two arms, the p arm (short arm) and the q arm (long arm). They are classified into four types based on the position of their centromeres: metacentric, submetacentric, acrocentric, and telocentric.

1.2.1 Metacentric chromosomes

Where the centromere is precisely situated at the center, dividing the chromosomes into two equal sections [chromosomes 1, 3, 16, 19, 20]. The two P and q arms are equally separated from the centromere and are referred to as m (**Figure 2**).

1.2.2 Sub metacentric chromosomes

Where the centromere is off-center on the chromosome [4, 5, 6, 7, 8, 9, 10, 11, 12, 17, 18, and X]. The shape of the sub metacentric chromosome is L, and it is labeled as sm. It contains unequal p and q arms (**Figure 2**).

1.2.3 Acrocentric chromosomes

Centromeres are generally found near the end of the chromosome, near the telomere [13, 14, 15, 21, 22, Y chromosome]. The p arm of the acrocentric chromosome contains nucleolar organizing regions that code for r RNA. Balanced and unbalanced translocations arise as a result of acrocentric chromosome centromeric region breakdown and fusion (**Figure 2**).

1.2.4 Telocentric chromosomes

The human genome contains no telomeric chromosomes. In mouse anaphase, telocentric chromosomes are generated predominantly. If only one arm is detected on the telocentric chromosome (**Figure 2**).

Non-disjunction of chromosomes occurs during meiotic and mitotic cell division (that is, inappropriate separation of sister chromatids during anaphase of meiosis I, II, and mitosis, resulting in an aberrant number of chromosomes, which leads to abnormalities). This nondisjunction is caused by inactive enzymes such as topoisomerase and helicase (binds sister chromatids in anaphase) [5].

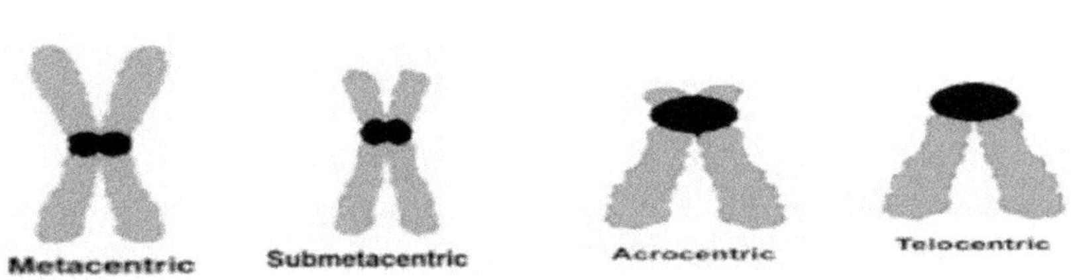

Figure 2.
Representation of metacentric, sub metacentric, acrocentric and telocentric chromosomes.

2. Diagnosis

There are some conventional and commonly used methods or techniques for detecting chromosomal abnormalities. The following are the four most popular techniques:

1. Karyotyping

2. Fluorescent InSitu Hybridization (FISH)

3. Chromosomal microarray

4. Quantitative Fluorescent – Polymerase Chain Reaction (QF- PCR).

2.1 Karyotyping

Karyotyping is a laboratory procedure that is used to diagnose chromosomal abnormalities both numerical and structural as well as related disorders. Samples for karyotyping can be peripheral blood, cord blood, bone marrow, amniotic fluid, or tissues. Lymphocytes are cultured in a medium and metaphase is arrested by the addition of colchicine. Later, the cells are treated with a hypotonic solution and fixed (3:1 methanol: acetic acid) on a glass slide with Carnoy's fixative before staining the chromosomes with Giemsa.

There are numerous banding techniques available for chromosomal distinction and arrangement; the most commonly used banding technique is GTG- banding. Based on the size, position of the centromere, and banding patterns, heterochromatin regions are AT rich and are darkly stained, while euchromatin regions have light bands. Chromosomes are reported in accordance with the standard nomenclature scheme (ISCN-International System for Human Cytogenomic Nomenclature) 2020. The total number of autosomes is mentioned first, followed by commas (,) and sex chromosomes in the description of human karyotype. The + and – signs represents the gain and loss of chromosomes.

If chromosomes are structurally rearranged or aberrant, structural designations such as del, dup, inv., and so on are used, and the structurally altered chromosomal numbering is given in brackets. If the rearrangement occurs inside or between two chromosomes, it is separated by a semicolon (;), male patient with Down syndrome and inversion 9 is stated as 47, XY, +21,inv(9). If the karyotype comprises mosaicism, two distinct cell lines are designated: 47, XY,+21,inv(9)/46,XY. Microdeletions, duplications and insertions which are smaller than 5 Mb in size, cannot be detected by the method of karyotyping has its own limitations. It does not recognize both homozygosity and loss of heterozygosity [6]. Infertility, primary amenorrhea, developmental delay, mental impairment, Hematological cancers, Fragile X syndrome, and other frequent disorders that necessitate chromosomal analysis. Limitations of Karyotyping can be fulfilled by next advanced tests like FISH and Microarray.

2.2 FISH

Fluorescent insitu hybridization is a technique that uses fluorescence probes to localize a portion of DNA, which then attaches to a specific target region that can be observed using a fluorescent microscope.

There are three types of probes used in FISH diagnostics:

2.2.1 Locus specific probes

These probes locate a specific gene on a specific chromosome.

2.2.2 Whole chromosome probe

Where numerous smaller samples and various tints of fluorescent dyes, each probe binds to a specific segment of the chromosome, resulting in a chromosomal map. As a result, any abnormality, such as translocation, can be immediately noticed.

2.2.3 Centromeric repeat probes

The number of chromosomes was determined by a repeating binding sequence. It is widely used in prenatal diagnosis, minor chromosomal abnormalities, and malignancy differential diagnosis. The main advantage of FISH is that it minimizes the Turn Around Time (TAT), which is specific for recognizing minor chromosomal abnormalities, and it can also detect the proportion of mosaicism.

2.3 Chromosomal microarray

Chromosomal microarray is a cost-effective and high-resolution prenatal test, which is based on alterations in the genome, or copy number variations. It is capable of detecting the entire chromosome on a single microchip. It primarily looks for microdeletions, duplications, and aneuploidy. According to the International standard Cytogenomic array consortium, chromosomal microarray is a commonly utilized tool in prenatal diagnostics. It is one of the tools for detecting Cytogenomic imbalances that has been revolutionized in the present era of Cytogenomic. Identification of DNA copy number gains and losses aids in the diagnosis and treatment of a variety of hereditary disorders.

2.4 QF-PCR

Quantitative fluorescence-polymerase chain reaction (QF-PCR) is a prenatal diagnostic molecular technology used to detect chromosomal aneuploidies such as 13,18,21 and sex chromosomes. This is a rapid and more automated technique than FISH and Karyotyping since no fetal cells are cultured. DNA can be extracted from amniotic fluid, tissue, or chronic villus samples, and fluorescent primers are used for analysis. It is inexpensive, quick, Faster and only a small amount of the sample is required for diagnosis. It is more robust and requires less labor and time than other traditional procedures such as Karyotyping and FISH.

3. Chromosomal abnormalities

Chromosomal abnormalities are grossly divided into numerical abnormalities and structural abnormalities.

3.1 Numerical abnormalities

Numeric abnormalities caused by the loss or gain of one or more chromosomes, which can be aneuploidy or polyploidy.

3.1.1 Aneuploidies

The gain or loss of chromosome is also known as aneuploidy. When a single chromosome is removed from a pair of chromosomes called monosomy [7]. Trisomy or tetrasomy occurs when one or more chromosomes are gained. It can occur either in Autosomal or sex chromosomes. Down syndrome, Edward syndrome, and Patau's syndrome are autosomal aneuploidies, while Klinefelter syndrome, Jacob syndrome (XYY), and Turner syndrome are sex chromosomal Aneuploidies (**Figure 3**).

3.1.2 Polyploidy

It is a condition in which a normal diploid cell gains one or more sets of chromosomes. Polyploidy occurs as a result of chromosomal disjunction during mitosis and meiosis which are typically observed in plants and animals and are not seen in humans. These syndromes are associated with a variety of phenotypical problems such as developmental delay, recurrent miscarriages, infertility, congenital heart abnormalities, and so on. Triploidy is an uncommon disorder in which a complete haploid set of additional chromosomes is present, resulting in miscarriage or premature death. Tetraploidy is a condition where cell contains four sets of chromosomes which are infrequent and resulting in spontaneous abortions.

3.1.2.1 Autosome aneuploidies

The common autosomal aneuploidies are described below.

3.1.2.2 Down syndrome (DS)

DS is the most frequent chromosomal anomaly caused by the inheritance of an additional chromosome 21. Down syndrome manifests itself in a variety of ways, some of which are listed below.

1. Non-disjunction of chromosomes: This occurs during gamete development i.e., during meiosis the pair of chromosomes 21 in egg or sperm fails to separate (**Figure 4A**).

2. Chromosome 21 splits and attaches to another chromosome in a Robertsonian translocation (**Figure 4B**).

3. Mosaicism is a term used to describe the pattern of where few cells show normal chromosomes set while some cells show extra chromosome 21.

DS is a complex genetic disease that is compatible with human post-term survival, and it is the most common survivable autosomal aneuploidy. It is difficult since chromosome 21 has over 200 protein-coding genes that can have direct and indirect effects on homeostasis in cells, tissues, organs, and systems [8].

Clinical features: DS is characterized by a protruding tongue, peculiar fingerprints, pelvic dysplasia, low set ears, a short neck, chinkey eyes, a sandal gap, mental retardation, epicanthic skin folds, and congenital heart disease in more than half of patients. Down syndrome patients have a high copy number of genes on chromosome 21, which causes gene overexpression and phenotypic abnormalities. Prenatal diagnosis for Down syndrome: Ultrasound for nuchal translucency, Quad screen, Amniocentesis or CVS.

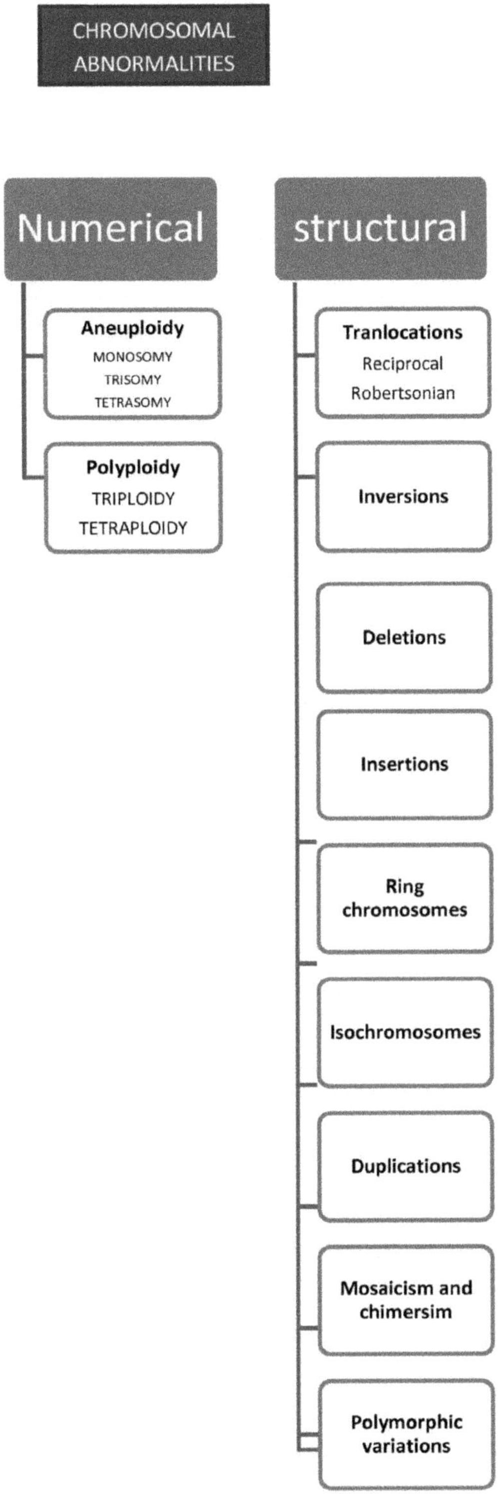

Figure 3.
Types of both numerical and structural abnormalities of chromosomes.

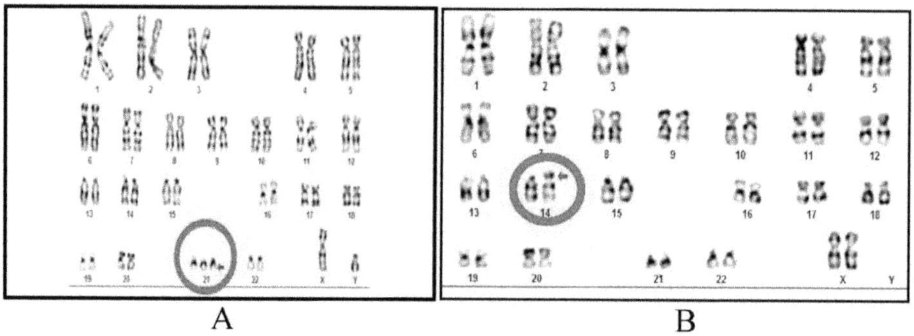

Figure 4.
Karyotype with 47, XY+21 indicating a free trisomy (A) and 46, XX rob t (14, 21); (q10;q10) indicating Robertsonian translocation.

Treatment/management: There is no specific cure for DS, however it can be managed through a comprehensive approach. Karyotyping is critical for establishing a diagnosis of DS and evaluating the syndrome's recurrence risk in following generations. To improve quality of life, DS should be addressed by a variety of specialists, including endocrinologists, cardiologists, audiologists, nutritionists, clinical geneticists/medical geneticists, and nutritionists [9]. DS patients need also get therapies such as occupational, speech, behavioral, and physical therapies in order to improve motor and communication abilities as well as manage or reduce behavioral difficulties, allowing them to live a normal social life.

3.1.2.3 Edward syndrome (ES)

Trisomy 18 is another term for ES (47, XY + 18 in males and 47XX + 18 in females), (**Figure 5**) named after the geneticist Edward who reported it, is caused by an extra copy of chromosome 18 caused by nondisjunction of meiotic gametes in sperm or egg. It mostly impacts fetal development and organogenesis.

Phenotypical characters: ES is characterized by microcephaly, cleft lip and palate, lung malformation, hypoplasia of skeletal muscles, growth retardation,

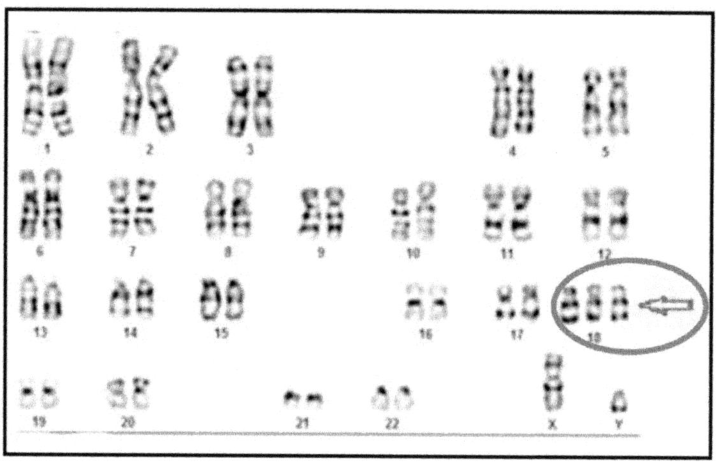

Figure 5.
Karyotype demonstrating trisomy 18 (47, XY, +18).

dysmorphic skull, cryptorchidism, neurodevelopmental delay, ventricular sept defects, low set ears, and other characteristics.

Treatment/management: There is no definitive treatment or management for children with trisomy 18, and there are ethical concerns because the condition has a high mortality rate. Because of its varying presentation, management focuses on correcting abnormalities and performing corrective operations as required.

3.1.2.4 Patau syndrome (PS)

PS, also known as trisomy 13 (47XY, +13 in males and 47XX,13 + in females) (**Figure 6**), is caused by an extra copy of chromosome 13 caused by nondisjunction and mosaicism. In comparison to other syndromes, the survival rate is lower.

Clinical features: Include cleft palate, polydactyly, and cranial deformities, as well as severe neurological abnormalities, ventricular septal defects, and seizures.

Treatment/management: Unfortunately, trisomy 13 has no known cure. It includes a variety of therapy and corrective operations based on the symptoms. Patients with cardiac defects may require cardiac surgery interventions, as well as other surgeries such as cleft lip repair, feeding tube placement, or corrective pediatrics or orthopedic surgeries, the use of hearing aids, specialized dietary feed, seizure prophylaxis, and urinary tract infection prevention antibodies.

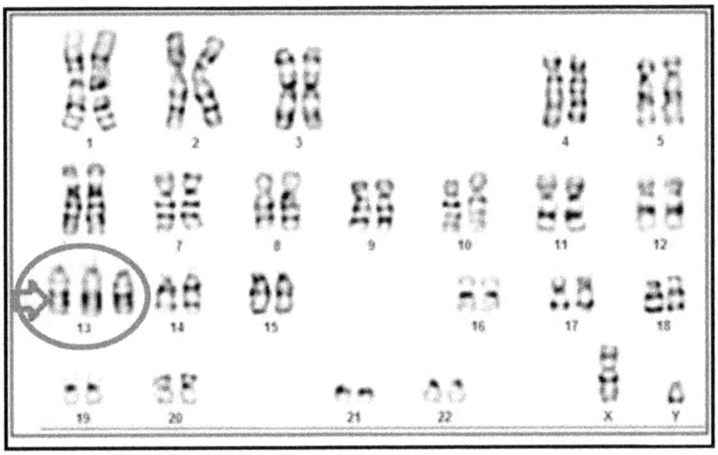

Figure 6.
Patau syndrome or trisomy 13 is indicated by the karyotype showing 47, XY, +13.

3.1.3. Allosome aneuploidies

3.1.3.1 Turners syndrome (TS)

TS is present in females and is caused by a total loss (45, X) (**Figure 7**) or partial loss of the X chromosome (deletion of the p arm 46, X, del (Xp), or isochromosome of the q arm), primarily due to a failure in the inheritance of the X chromosome from male paternal origin. Turner syndrome is frequently mosaic, with 45XO/46XX indicating the presence of two distinct cell lines.

Clinical features: Turner syndrome women have short stature, delayed puberty, a webbed neck, puffiness in the hands and feet, a congenital cardiac defect, and

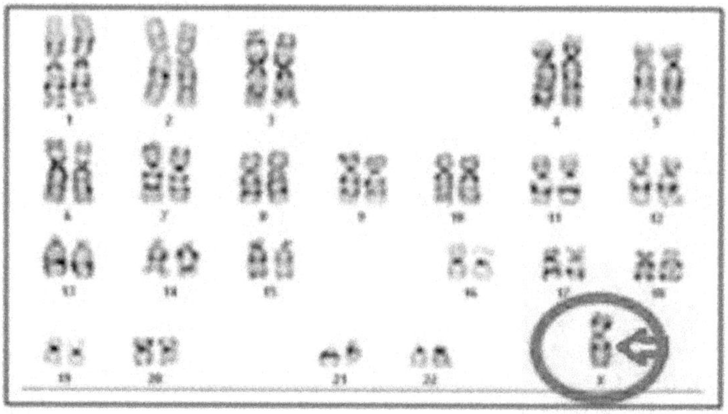

Figure 7.
Karyotype 45, XO, indicating Turner syndrome.

infertility. Women with hypogonadotropic hypogonadism and undeveloped ovaries may benefit from hormone treatment, which may aid in the development of secondary sexual characteristics. Affected individuals are at a significant risk of developing autoimmune illnesses, type 2 diabetes, and renal abnormalities [10].

Treatment and management: TS is primarily treated or managed with hormonal therapy, such as injections of human growth hormone in the early stages of life to increase height. Hormone replacement therapy, such as estrogen, is used to faster the development of secondary sexual characteristics. Uterus transplantation is a recent advancement in treatment that is well-established in developed countries.

3.1.3.2 Klinefelter syndrome (KS)

KS is most common in men who have an additional X chromosome, resulting in a karyotype of 47, XXY (**Figure 8**). Incomplete meiotic division in gametes, such as egg or sperm, results in an extra copy of the X chromosome. There will be more than two copies of the X chromosome in some uncommon and severe situations, resulting in the karyotype 48XXXY, 49XXXXY. Another type of mosaic Klinefelter in which the intensity of symptoms may be reduced is mosaic Klinefelter.

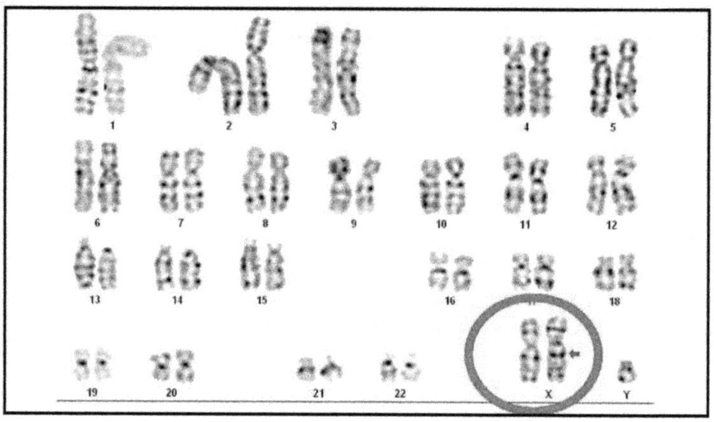

Figure 8.
Karyotype 47,XXY indicates Klinefelter syndrome.

Clinical features: Individuals with this syndrome may have delayed mildestones, taller than average, have longer legs and shorter toes, have delayed or incomplete puberty, urogenital abnormalities, weak bones, gynecomastia (breast enlargement), hormonal imbalances, intellectual difficulty, and infertility.

Treatment/management: Hormone treatment in childhood may improve brain and neurological development. In cases of infertility, depending on the count and morphology of the sperm, assisted reproductive procedures such as Intra Cytoplasmic Sperm Injection (ICSI) may be a viable alternative [11].

3.1.3.3 Jacob syndrome (XYY) or XYY Syndrome

It is a unique sex chromosomal disorder in which people have an extra Y chromosome due to nondisjunction in meiotic II division and is only seen in males. This extra Y chromosome is the result of father's erroneous spermatogenesis. Jacob syndrome (XYY) [12] has the karyotype 47, XYY (**Figure 9**).

Clinical features: Tallness, muscle weakness, hypertonia, ADHD (Attention deficit hyperactivity disorder), altered testosterone, congenital cardiac problems, neurological abnormalities, and a curled pennis are all symptoms of this condition. This syndrome is associated with a significant incidence of asthma and seizures, and symptoms vary from case to case. Individuals with this syndrome are more likely to be infertile.

Treatment/management: Jacob syndrome (XYY) is treated symptomatically and supportively. Speech therapy, occupational therapy, or school-based learning disability support may be effective. Individuals with this condition are usually quite amenable to early diagnosis and therapy. Other behavioral difficulties are addressed in accordance with their severity. Individuals with attention deficit and hyperactivity disorder, as well as difficulty with social interactions and in certain severe cases they may face suicidal tendencies also.

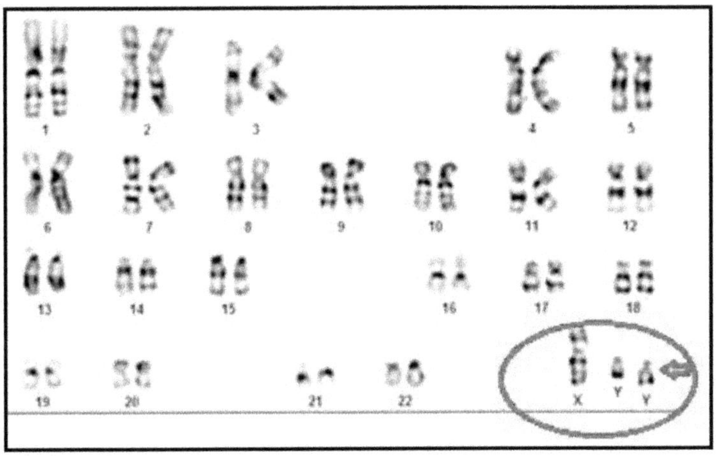

Figure 9.
Karyotype showing 47, XYY indicating Jacob Syndrome or XYY Syndrome.

3.2 Structural abnormalities

Structural abnormalities are caused by structural changes such as inappropriate joining or breaking of chromosomal segments and rearrangement of chromosomal segments, which results in incorrect lengths of the p and q arms of a chromosome. There is a chromosomal material exchange that modifies chromosome structure with no loss of genetic material. Unbalanced rearrangement occurs when a portion of a chromosome is removed or lost. When compared to unbalanced chromosomal changes, balanced chromosomal changes are anticipated to have less of an impact because genetic information is retained. Infertility, spontaneous pregnancy loss, and hematological malignancies are all linked to structural defects. Translocations, inversions, deletions, insertions, ring chromosomes, isochromosomes, duplications, mosaicism, chimerism, and polymorphic variations are some of the major structural abnormalities (**Figure 3**).

3.2.1 Translocations

Translocations are defined as the rearrangement of chromosomes/segments between non-homologous chromosomes which have no genetic material loss or gain. These are divided into two types (**Table 1**):

1. Reciprocal translocation (Balanced).

2. Robertsonian translocation.

3.2.1.1 Reciprocal translocations

Where there is a translocation or exchange of parts from two separate chromosomes (**Figure 10**). Inheritance of translocation occurs when one parent has derived chromosomes and the other parent has a normal pair of chromosomes, resulting in three sorts of chromosomal passing possibilities:

- they can pass both normal chromosomes,
- one normal and another derivative,
- two derivative chromosomes.

S. no	Type of chromosomal abnormalities	Karyotypes
1.	Numerical abnormality -	
	Monosomy (Turner syndrome)	45,XO
	Trisomies- Edward syndrome Patau syndrome Down syndrome	47,XX +18/47,XY +18 47, XX+13/47, XY+21 47, XX+21/47, XY+21
2.	Sex chromosomes abnormalities – Klinefelter syndrome Jacob syndrome	47,XXY 47,XYY
3.	Structural abnormalities such as translocations- Reciprocal translocations Robertsonian translocations Insertions Inversions Duplications Deletions Mosaicism Polymorphic variants Ring chromosomes	46,XX,t(4;12) 45,XY,t(14;21) 46 XX,ins9 46,XX, (inv9) (p12 q13) 46, XY, dup7 46, XX, 4p- 45, XO/46,XX 46,XX, 9qh+/Yqh+ 46,XX, r (21)

Table 1.
The type of chromosomal abnormalities and the karyotype notation.

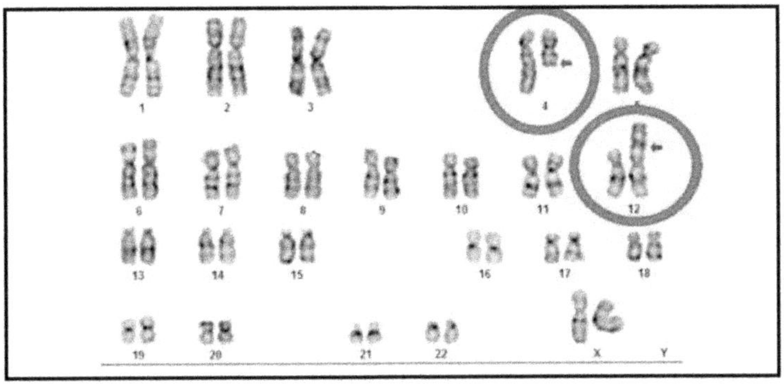

Figure 10.
Karyotype with 46,XX, t(4;12) demonstrating balanced reciprocal translocation among chromosomes 4 and 12.

The risk of translocation is proportional to the amount of chromosomal exchange, and it increases further when two defective chromosomes are received. De novo translocations are more perilous than inherited translocations. There may be multiple or triple reciprocal translocations at times [13].

3.2.1.2 Robertsonian translocation

This type of translocation occurs between (14, 15, 16, 21, 22) acrocentric chromosomes, in which one chromosome joins to another (D or G) (**Figure 11**). The fusion of two long arms of chromosomes 14 and 21 results in the translocated Downs syndrome phenotype. The presence of nucleolar organizing zones, satellite DNA (highly repetitive sequences), and r RNA sequences aids in the union of acrocentric centromeric regions, resulting in chromosome translocation. Parents with Robertsonian translocations have aberrant offspring due to incorrect meiotic division segregation. There is a greater likelihood that progeny will have abnormalities such as DS, PS, and so on. Carriers may exhibit a normal phenotype. Female carriers are more likely than male carriers to pass on the Down syndrome phenotype. Miscarriages, male infertility, and other complications result from Robertsonian translocation [14].

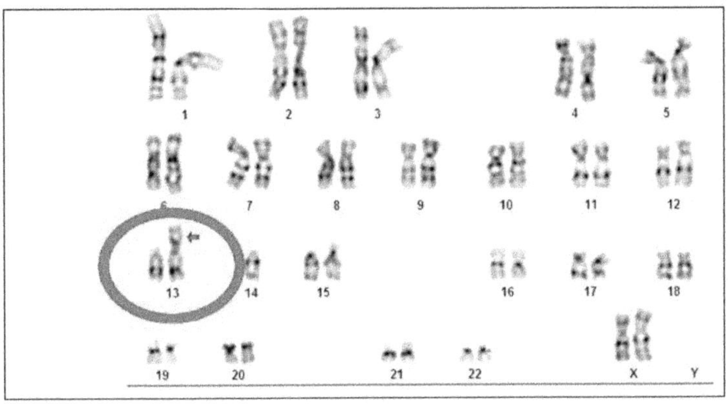

Figure 11.
A karyotype with 45, XX, rob t(13;14) indicating a Robertsonian translocation between 13 and 14 chromosomes.

3.2.2 Ring chromosomes

These are circular chromosomes, which result in the fusion of ends of a single chromosome due to a break in the terminal ends of both the p and q arms, resulting in some genetic material loss (**Figure 12**). Lilian Vaughan Morgan was the first to describe the ring chromosomes found in flies. The ring chromosome is denoted by the letter r and the chromosome number 46, XX, r(21) & 46, XY, r(1), etc., and it is a rare structural aberration [15]. Ring chromosome 14 and 20 syndrome is a common abnormality in epilepsy. The ring chromosome's phenotype is determined by the original deletion and instability caused by ring structure creation; there may be a loss or gain of certain secondary chromosome material, and carriers can be asymptomatic or cause major clinical symptoms. The majority of ring chromosome carriers are sterile. Cytogenetic studies such as karyotype and FISH demonstrate that ring chromosomes can be dicentric, interlocking, solitary, or multicentric. Because of the fragility of the ring structure during meiosis, inheritance is relatively uncommon in ring syndrome cases.

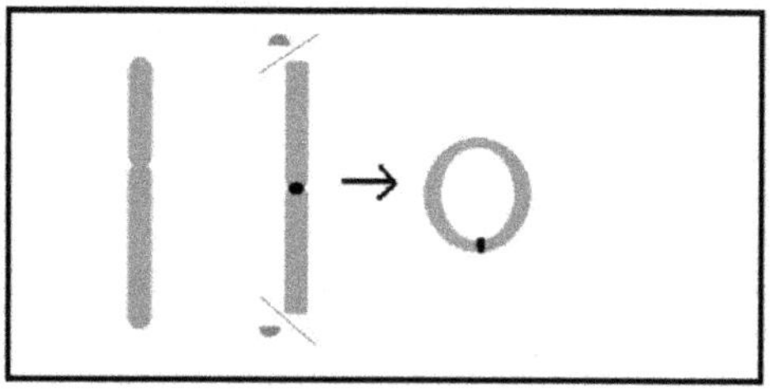

Figure 12.
Cartoon depicting the formation of a ring chromosome after breakage.

3.2.3 Inversions

Rearrangements of the same chromosome caused by reversal of gene order via breakage and reinsertion of fragment. Inversions are associated to reproductive difficulties such as recurrent pregnancy loss, infertility, position effect variation, and so on. Inversions can be classified as single inversion, complex inversion, homozygous inversion, or heterozygous inversion based on the segments and breaks. There are as follows (i) paracentric inversion and (ii) pericentric inversion.

3.2.3.1 Paracentric inversion

Inversions that occur within a single chromosome on a single arm without the participation of the centromere are classified as paracentric. During this process, chromosomes break and rearrange themselves by flipping 180 degrees. The effect of paracentric inversion is a loss of reproductive potential, and the chances of meiosis chromosome separation and alignment of non-inverted homologous chromosomes are reduced as a result of inversion, resulting in acentric or dicentric chromosomes, deletion of chromosomes, or sometimes balanced inversion in the case of even crossovers [16]. Because of the imbalanced chromosomal rearrangements, both men and women are at a significant risk of infertility (**Figure 13A**).

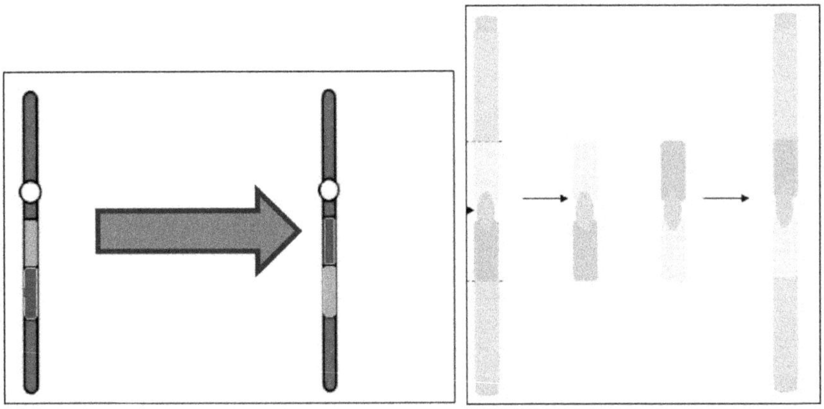

Figure 13.
Cartoon depicting paracentric inversion 13(A) and pericentric reverse 13(B).

3.2.3.2 Pericentric inversion

Inversion occurs when the centromere is involved, and there is a breakpoint on both arms and more frequently than paracentric inversion. Like paracentric inversion during meiosis chromatid separation, even crossings result in 50 percent balanced inversion and odd crossovers result in numerical abnormalities, which are aneuploidies caused by chromatid inversion, deletion, and duplication. One of the most prevalent examples of inversion is on chromosome 9, where the break point occurs between p arm p11 and long arm q 13. The female inversion 9 nomenclature is specified as 46,XX, (inv9) (p12 q13). Some of the most prevalent disorders associated with inversion 9 are Walker Warburg syndrome, newborn diabetes, and acute leukemia (**Figure 13B**).

3.2.4 Isochromosomes

Isochromosomes are defective chromosomes in which one chromosome has mirror images of a single chromosome arm, resulting in the loss of the other arm. Normal p and q arms will be present on the remaining homologous chromosome. Isochromes are created as a result of incorrect division, specifically U type strand division, which results in dicentric or bi centromeric chromosomes. Pallister-Killian syndrome, caused by isochromosome 12 p, and cat eye syndrome, produced by fusion of the short arm of chromosome 22 and on isochromosome 17q, are two syndromes related with isochromosomes [17].

3.2.5 Deletions

Deletions, which occur frequently spontaneously, result in the removal or fracture of a section from a chromosome, resulting in the loss of genetic material. One of the causes of deletion is exposure to radiations like as UV rays, X-rays, gamma rays, and so on. There are two categories of deletions; (1) *Interstitial deletion:* Deletion induced by two or more breaks in between the genes and (2) *Terminal deletion*: Deletion triggered by terminal ends (**Figure 14**). One typical example is cri du chat syndrome, which is caused by a deletion on the p 15.2 region of chromosome 5 [18]. Some deletions on chromosome 15 can be caused through inheritance from father and mother, such as Prader-Willi or Angelman syndrome (imprinting disorders).

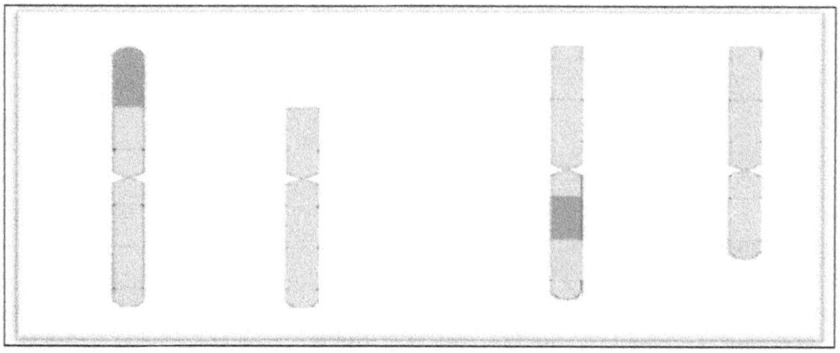

Figure 14.
Illustration of interstitial and terminal deletions on a chromosome.

3.2.6 Duplications

Duplication leads to the development of an extra copy of a chromosomal segment. Duplication does not pose a significant risk, but it does promote evolution. Some of the human genes produced by duplication through evolution are human globin genes; they arose from predecessors, some of which express in the embryonic stage and others in the adult stage [19]. Tandem duplication occurs when the duplicated gene is near to or contiguous to the original gene, whereas displaced duplication occurs when the duplicated region is far from the gene. *MECP2* duplication syndrome is a common occurrence in humans, particularly in men, and is caused by X chromosomal duplication. 7 q 11.23 duplication syndromes are another kind of duplication that causes numerous neurological phenotypic effects.

3.2.7 Polymorphic variants

Variants that occur in chromosomal heterochromatin regions. Variants in long arms are mainly found in the paracentric region of heterochromatin, and all acrocentric chromosomes have polymorphism. An increase or decrease in the lengths of chromosomes in the heterochromatin region can be represented by the symbols qh+, qh-., Polymorphic variations are a common anomaly reported in infertility and spontaneous miscarriages. They are regarded as normal because they have been identified in the general population. Yqh is the most prevalent polymorphic variation found in male infertility [20].

The most common polymorphic variants found in the long arm of chromosomes are 1qh+, 16qh+, 9qh+, and 1qh-, and short arm chromosome polymorphic variants are 14 ps+,15 ps+,13 ps+, and so on. These polymorphic variants can be identified using the silver NOR (Nucleolar Organizing Regions) banding technique (**Figure 15**).

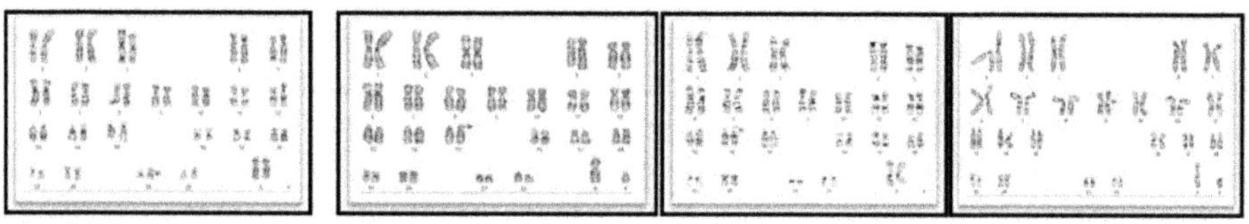

A) 46, XX, 21ps+ B) 46, XY, 15ps+ C) 46,XX,14ps+ D)46,XY,9qh+

Figure 15.
Karyotype indicating 46,XX,21 ps+,46,XY,15 ps+,46,XX,14 ps+ and 46,XY,9qh+ polymorphic variants on chromosome 21,14,15 and 9. (A) 46 XX, 21 ps+, (B) 46 XY, 15 ps+, (C) 46,XX,14 ps+, (D)46,XY,9qh+.

3.2.8 Mosaicism

Mosaicism occurs during the developmental process. During zygote formation, distinct cell lineages emerge, resulting in diverse genotypes in different cells. Some cells have a normal set of chromosomes, while others have abnormal chromosomes. Mosaicism is classified into two categories based on cell origin: germ line mosaicism and somatic mosaicism. Germ line mosaicism develops in germ cells when the individual carrying the germ cells is not deformed but the children are. In somatic cells, where somatic mosaicism occurs. Confined mosaicism occurs in a variety of organs. Mosaicism can be inherited or occur sporadically [21]. Some patients with mosaic versions of Ret syndrome, Down syndrome, Klinefelter syndrome, and Cornelia de Lange syndrome have a lower risk than others.

3.2.9 Chimerism

Chimerism differs from mosaicism in that two distinct genotypes are produced as a result of the embryonic fusing of two zygotes. It can be a tetra gametic chimera in which identical or non-identical twins' fuse, resulting in male, female, or bisexual characteristics. For the first time, Taylor Muhl found chimersim. Another sort of chimersim is blood group chimersim, which occurs when a person has two separate blood cell types.

3.2.10 Insertions

Insertion occurs when a chromosomal fragment gets inserted into another chromosome or inside the same chromosome in a non-adjacent area (**Figure 16**). Insertions can cause a massive chromosomal rearrangement with numerous phenotypic effects. These repercussions are primarily determined by the size and location of the chromosome. There are two kinds of insertions: intrachromosomal insertions and interchromosomal insertions. Individuals who are carriers of intrachromosomal insertions are more likely to have a child with an aberrant or unbalanced karyotype.

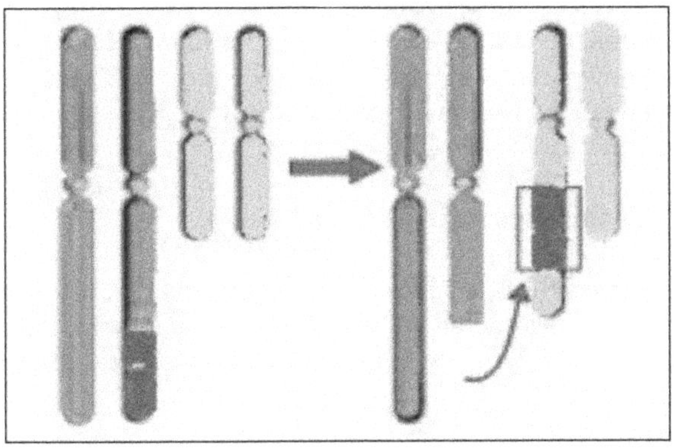

Figure 16.
Image representing insertion of chromosome segment.

3.3 Management and prevention

With the increasing incidence and prevalence of genetic conditions, it should be addressed and there is a need to focus and more attention towards the prevention of genetic conditions to reduce the global burden with syndromes or birth defects. The government should take the initiative, for preventive strategies and measures adopted in tertiary care institutions or hospitals.

3.3.1 Prenatal screening

Prenatal screening programs have a significant impact on improved pregnancy outcomes. Between 11 and 13 weeks of gestation, NT scan should be performed, as well as other biochemical markers such as a double, triple, and quatriple marker at the proper gestational ages. An altered marker or scan, in the case of a substantial family history, such as a prior child diagnosed with a genetic condition, invasive prenatal testing is recommended either by chronic villus sampling (CVS) or amniocentesis.

Chronic villus sampling (CVS) is an invasive procedure performed on a growing placenta between 11 and 14 weeks of gestation. Under ultrasound guidance, a needle with a syringe is inserted transabdominally based on the position of the placenta, after which the tissue is removed and inspected. Based on the indication, the excised tissue was subjected to FISH and Karyotyping, Chromosomal microarray, or advanced molecular testing.

Amniocentesis is another invasive method performed by a professional radiologist between the gestational ages of 16 and 20 weeks after informed consent, in which a needle is introduced to aspirate amniotic fluid. Regardless of the prenatal diagnosis following CVS or amniocentesis, each individual has their own emotional, psychological, economical, and religious reasons for continuing the pregnancy or deciding for a medical termination in the event of abnormalities to decrease burden with the advent of genomics. Genetic testing for preimplantation embryos is being developed.

3.3.2 Pre-implantation genetic testing (PGT)

Is a genetic test that is conducted on embryos during IVF prior to implantation in the uterus. The term *PGT-A* involves the detection of Aneuploidies in all chromosomes whereas *PGT-SR* identifies structural rearrangements in all chromosomes such as translocations, inversions etc. *PGT-M* is for identification of a single gene condition with a known diagnosis in the family history. PGT is typically chosen for patients with advanced maternal age, recurrent pregnancy losses, and a strong family history of genetic disorders.

3.4 Implications of chromosomal abnormalities

Some common conditions, such as primary amenorrhea, infertility, recurrent pregnancy loss, syndromes such as Down, Edward, Patau, and hematological malignancies, are connected or associated with chromosomal abnormalities.

3.4.1 Primary amenorrhea

It is a condition in which females of reproductive age are unable to achieve menarche and lack certain secondary sexual characteristics. This is caused by monosomy X (45,XO) or isochromosome X or partial deletion on X chromosome, as well as other chromosomal abnormalities such as ring chromosome X. Following confirmation of diagnosis via karyotyping or FISH, appropriate care, such as hormonal therapy and subsequent ART (Assisted Reproductive Techniques) recommendations are elucidated.

3.4.2 Primary and secondary infertility

Primary infertility refers to the inability to conceive after two year of unprotected intercourse, whereas secondary infertility is inability to sustain to term pregnancy. These may be due to chromosomal abnormalities, hormone imbalances, anatomical inabilities, and other factors. One of the most common chromosomal abnormalities associated with infertility are Turner, Klinefelter, Swyer syndrome and translocations.

3.4.3 Recurrent pregnancy loss

The most common reason of recurrent pregnancy losses (RPL) is chromosomal abnormalities. Balanced translocations, inversions and polymorphic variants are commonly observed in RPL. Maternal age is one of the risk factors for recurrent pregnancy loss, which increases the incidence of trisomies.

3.4.4 Syndromes

Most of the common genetic syndromes are caused due to numerical and structural chromosomal abnormalities. DS is caused gain of chromosome 21, TS is due to monosomy X and Cri du chat is caused due to partial deletion on the chromosome 5 respectively. These syndromes are associated with clinical features like developmental delay, speech difficulties, hearing impairment, feeding difficulties, cardiac defects and intellectual disability.

3.4.5 Malignancies

Identification of chromosomal abnormalities is useful in the diagnosis, treatment, management, and prognosis of several hematological and solid malignancies. Specific chromosomal abnormalities can help in the differential diagnosis and therapy planning of various malignancies. Balanced translocations, inversions, partial deletions, trisomies, and other chromosomal abnormalities are common in hematological malignancies. Some of the translocations seen in acute myeloid leukemia are t (8:21) and t(9:22) in chronic myeloid leukemia, both of which result in the proliferation of numerous myeloid lineages. In the case of primary MDS, del 5q and del 7q, as well as translocations such as t(11:16) and t(3:21), have been often reported. Some structural rearrangements have a strong relationship with clinical and morphological characteristics.

4. Conclusion

Identification of Chromosomal abnormalities plays an immense role in the diagnosis, treatment/management, risk assessment, extended family screening and it also helps in taking appropriate informed decisions. Increasing awareness and implementation of certain genetic testing policies in the health care sector helps in prevention and control of genetic diseases.

Author details

Subhadra Poornima[1*], Saranya Vadrevu[1] and Imran Ali Khan[2]

1 Department of Genetics and Molecular Medicine, Kamineni Life Sciences, Moula-ali, Hyderabad, India

2 Department of Clinical Laboratory Sciences, College of Applied Medical Sciences, King Saud University, Riyadh, Saudi Arabia

*Address all correspondence to: subhadrapoornima1@gmail.com

References

[1] Parmar JJ, Padinhateeri R. Nucleosome positioning and chromatin organization. Curr Opin Struct Biol. 2020;64:111-118.

[2] Baldi S, Korber P, Becker PB. Beads on a string—nucleosome array arrangements and folding of the chromatin fiber. Nature structural & molecular biology. 2020;27(2):109-118.

[3] Chen X, Yang H, Liu G, Zhang Y. NUCOME: A comprehensive database of nucleosome organization referenced landscapes in mammalian genomes. BMC bioinformatics. 2021;22(1):1-15.

[4] Talbert PB, Henikoff S. What makes a centromere? Experimental cell research. 2020;389(2):1-13.

[5] Shindo N, Otsuki M, Uchida KS, Hirota T. Prolonged mitosis causes separase deregulation and chromosome nondisjunction. Cell Reports. 2021;34(3):108652.

[6] Levy B. Prenatal Diagnosis of Chromosomal Abnormalities: From Karyotype to Microarray. Genetic Disorders and the Fetus. 2021:547-571.

[7] Yahaya TO, Oladele EO, Anyebe D, Obi C, Bunza M, Sulaiman R, et al. Chromosomal abnormalities predisposing to infertility, testing, and management: a narrative review. Bulletin of the National Research Centre. 2021;45(1):1-15.

[8] Antonarakis SE, Skotko BG, Rafii MS, Strydom A, Pape SE, Bianchi DW, et al. Down syndrome. Nature Reviews Disease Primers. 2020;6(1):1-20.

[9] Alsahabi I, Alobaidi A, Alahmari AS, Almohsen N, Alhamoud AH. Clinical presentation and successful management of an infant with Down syndrome and COVID-19 in Riyadh, Saudi Arabia. Cureus. 2021;13(2):1-3.

[10] Yusrawati Y, Putri DM. A Case of Prenatal Diagnosis of Turner Syndrome with Ultrasonography. Andalas Obstetrics And Gynecology Journal. 2021;5(1):119-129.

[11] Bonomi M, Rochira V, Pasquali D, Balercia G, Jannini E, Ferlin A. Klinefelter Italia NG. 2017. Klinefelter syndrome (KS): genetics, clinical phenotype and hypogonadism Journal Endocrinolology Investigation. 40:123-34.

[12] Chen Y, Lai Y, Xu F, Qin H, Tang Y, Huang X, Meng L, Su J, Sun W, Shen Y, Wei H. The application of expanded noninvasive prenatal screening for genome-wide chromosomal abnormalities and genetic counseling. The Journal of Maternal-Fetal & Neonatal Medicine. 2021 30:1-7.

[13] Chakraborty A, Palo I, Roy S, Koh SW, Hande MP, Banerjee B. A Novel Balanced Chromosomal Translocation in an Azoospermic Male: A Case Report. Journal of Reproduction & Infertility. 2021;22(2):133-137.

[14] Poornima, S., Swarnalatha Daram, R. K., & Hasan, Q. (2020). Robertsonian and balanced reciprocal translocation in both child and mother with a history of recurrent abortions. Journal of reproduction & infertility, *21*(1):61-67.

[15] Pristyazhnyuk IE, Menzorov AG. Ring chromosomes: from formation to clinical potential. Protoplasma. 2018;255(2):439-449.

[16] Durmaz E, Kerdaffrec E, Katsianis G, Kapun M, Flatt T. How Selection Acts on Chromosomal Inversions. eLS. 2020 Sep 30;1:307-315.

[17] Koczkodaj D, Muzyka-Kasietczuk J, Chocholska S, Podhorecka M. Prognostic significance of

isochromosome 17q in hematologic malignancies. Oncotarget. 2021 Mar 30;12(7):708-718.

[18] Lokmanoğlu BN, Mutlu A, Livanelioğlu A, Haliloğlu G. The general movements assessment and effects of an early intervention in an infant with Cri du chat syndrome: a case report. The Turkish Journal of Pediatrics. 2021;63(1):167-173.

[19] Dennis MY, Harshman L, Nelson BJ, Penn O, Cantsilieris S, Huddleston J, et al. The evolution and population diversity of human-specific segmental duplications. Nature ecology & evolution. 2017;1(3):1-10.

[20] Hong Y, Zhou Y-W, Tao J, Wang S-X, Zhao X-M. Do polymorphic variants of chromosomes affect the outcome of in vitro fertilization and embryo transfer treatment? Human Reproduction. 2011;26(4):933-940.

[21] Milani DAQ, Chauhan PR. Genetics, Mosaicism. StatPearls [Internet]. 2020:1-9.

CPSIA information can be obtained
at www.ICGtesting.com
Printed in the USA
LVHW060757130422
716078LV00006B/224

9 781839 693649